APPLYING TO MEDICAL SCHOOL
for the NON-TRADITIONAL STUDENT

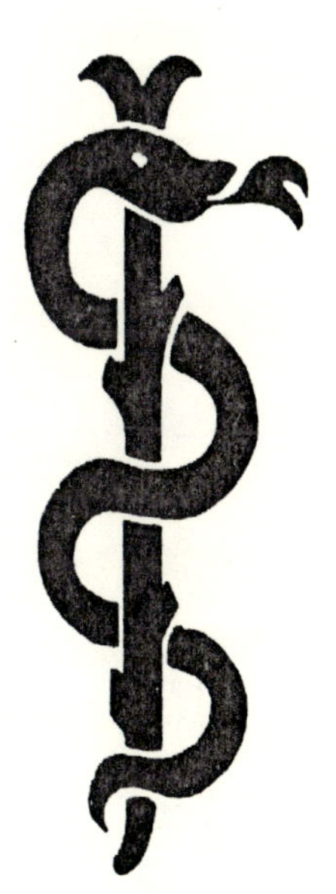

From Decision to Admission—

Interviews

with

Successful

Applicants

by Bryan Goss

I would like to take this opportunity
to thank each of the individuals
who I interviewed and
all of the other people who
helped make this project happen.

Thank you,
Bryan Goss
Second Year Medical Student
Northwestern Medical School

Author: Bryan Goss

Editors: Peter Goss, Bryan Goss

Cover design and layout: Beverly Goss

Poetry Contribution (Page 201) : Wesley Hilger

Copyright Counsel: Hunter Farrell
Transcription: Lorena Shih, Troy Foster

Lakeshore–Pearson Publications
Send questions or comments to:
bgoss@nwu.edu

Introduction

I decided to write this book while I was a non-traditional pre-med student who was going through the application process. I searched for a book that addressed the non-traditional student. Many other books that I did read on the subject of getting into medical school were helpful, but none gave me personal accounts of different non-traditional students who had been through the process of applying to medical school themselves.

This book employs an interview format because what each individual reader will get out of it depends on that individual's needs at the time. Also, the interview style allows each interviewee to expand on meaningful and personal accounts from their application process. Each person answers questions chosen to encompass the period of time from before the individual decided to go back to school up to the time of his or her acceptance to medical school.

The first two questions pertain to the interviewee's background and to their personal decision to go back to school and then apply to medical school. The reader should be able to identify with one or more of the students and be able to say " hey, this person has a similar personal and professional background to me" and therefore have an example of a successful applicant with a similar background.

The next few questions address the courses and the type of premedical program that the interviewee enrolled in, which include traditional college, night school, and specific post -bacc. premedical programs. Additional questions identify strategies for choosing courses, choosing teachers, and taking classes while working. Subsequent questions address specific study habits and strategies for achieving success in premedical course work.

I include   questions on advisement   to illustrate the avenues at each school which make the process of medical school application and class advisement easier. Many of the stories will allow others to avoid the problems that these individuals experienced.

Another important part of the medical school selection process is involvement in the medical community and other activities that make for a well rounded individual. The answers to these questions detail the types of activities that successful applicants participate in. Not surprisingly, there is a large variety in both activity and time commitment.

Next, were questions pertaining to the MCAT(Medical College Admissions Test.) Interviewees answer specific questions about when to take the test, how to study for the test and how long to study for the test. There was a great variety of answers to these questions for many reasons including personal aptitude, work schedule, and other time commitments.

The standardized medical school application, or AMCAS, is required by the majority of medical schools. The application consists of a one page essay as well as a non-essay section. The space on the form is extremely limited and forces most post bacc. students to pick and chose what will make the final draft. Some suggestions are made in the interviewee's answers. The AMCAS essay or personal statement usually requires extensive time to prepare and the interviews offer suggestions on content and subject matter.

When the AMCAS application is received favorably by a medical school admission committee, a secondary application will be requested, which requires the applicant to write additional essays (and send in more money) to the school. The interviewees discuss an organized approach to these applications. Furthermore, the students address how, when and if additional information should be sent to the schools after the formal application.

Most of the interviewed students state that timing of the medical school application is extremely important. They discuss strategies to complete the application professionally, quickly, and thoroughly. However, all the students did not agree.

Most applicants cannot apply to all available medical schools, so the decisions regarding which and how many schools to apply to must be made. Interviewees speak about the number of schools each applied to and discuss the reasons for applying to the schools that they chose.

Recommendations are required of each applicant to medical school. These recommendations are important and can greatly influence acceptance or rejection for medical school. The interviewed students discuss why they chose specific professors and employers, which should aid the applicant in the process of choosing recommenders.

If the application , class grades, and recommendations are favorably received by the admissions committee the applicant will be invited for an interview. The medical students discuss different interviewing styles and the questions asked . Readers should also be attentive to the student's advice on interview preparation.

The light at the end of the tunnel is acceptance to medical

school. Once accepted, students have the pleasurable decision of selecting where they will spend the next four years. Each interview ends with closing thoughts and advice from each of the medical students.

Individuals Interviewed

THERESE LUCIETTO: Therese is twenty-nine, married, with one daughter. She received a Bachelor of Science degree in Engineering from Northwestern University. She then worked as a materials engineer in industry.

HOWARD HORNE: Howard is forty-one years old and married. He spent the majority of his career working for the New York City Emergency Medical Services culminating as the Associate Director of Service. Additionally, he has worked as a consultant in public health and asset management. Howard received his undergraduate degree as well as a Master of Public Health from the University of Pennsylvania.

JOANNE ZELL: Joanne is twenty-seven. She graduated from Michigan University with a degree in Psychology. After college she worked as a National Parks Ranger at the Grand Canyon and later as a counselor for emotionally disturbed children.

SANDEEP DAVE: Sandeep is twenty-seven years old. He received an undergraduate degree in India and subsequently a Master of Biomedical Engineering Degree at Northwestern University. Prior to medical school, he worked as a systems analyst.

MARGY AITKEN: Margy is twenty-nine years old. She worked as a professional medical illustrator and creative director for a medical chart company and later ran her own business as a free-lance medical illustrator. She received her undergraduate and Master of Medical Illustration Degrees from Michigan University.

LISA STRANC: Lisa is twenty-eight years old. She majored in Psychology and graduated from Loyola University while working full time.

STEVE HERWICK: Steve is twenty-seven years old. He graduated from Northwestern University with a degree in Political Science. He then worked as a marketing and fund-raising manager for the Museum of Broadcast Journalism in Chicago..

ARTURO GUTIERREZ: Arturo is twenty-nine and married. After graduating from Cornell University with an Engineering degree he worked as an engineer for two years. Later, he worked as a product management executive in consumer products, pharmaceuticals, and candy.

SUSAN LIBMAN: Susan is thirty two and married. She graduated from Stanford with a degree in Political Science. After college, she worked in sales and marketing for a medical equipment company.

ALLISON MANGURTEN: Allison is a twenty-seven years old. She graduated from the University of Illinois, Champaign-Urbana, with a degree in Business Administration. After college, she worked as a CPA for a public accounting firm.

WILLIAM MCCULLOUGH: Bill is married and thirty-one years old. His undergraduate degree is in Computer Science from Purdue University . Before coming to medical school, he spent eight years in the U.S. Navy as a line officer. He also has a Master's in Business Administration.

HEIDI MEMMEL: Heidi is twenty seven years old. She graduated from Northwestern University with a degree in German Studies. Before medical school she worked for an executive recruiting firm as research manager and executive recruiter in the petroleum industry.

ELISABETH WEIL: Elizabeth is forty years old. She graduated from Colorado College in 1978. After working for a number of years, she went back to graduate school at Northwestern and received a master's degree in Speech Pathology in 1984. After graduating, she practiced as a speech pathologist for two years in Florida and then at the Rehabilitation Institute of Chicago.

LISA BERG: Lisa is thirty and married. She graduated from University of Wisconsin at Eau Claire with a Bachelor of Science in Nursing. She then worked as a bone marrow transplant nurse in a number of hospitals.

MICHELLE MONTPETIT: Michelle is a twenty six years old. She graduated from Drake University with a degree in Pharmacy and worked as a in-patient pharmacist at Northwestern Hospital before applying to medical school. She continues to work during medical school as time permits.

Interview One — Therese Lucietto

THERESE LUCIETTO: Therese is twenty-nine, married, with one daughter. She received a Bachelor of Science degree in Engineering from Northwestern University. She then worked as a materials engineer in industry.

Q.
Tell me a little of your education and other interests before you came to medical school.

A:
I have a Bachelor of Science in Material Science in Engineering from Northwestern University in Evanston. I graduated in 1989. I was a traditional student up until that point. When I graduated I started working. I had also started working on master's degree courses because I was not positive of exactly what I wanted to do. I pursued a master's degree in electronic materials and surface science and also ceramics and I completed most of the course work with the exception of the master's thesis which I still have time to complete but I doubt I will.

Right after I graduated in 1989, I married.   My husband was in school going part-time. He had gone part-time on and off for about 10 years and he earned a Bachelor of Science in Electrical Engineering.

I worked full-time until the summer of 1990 when I was able to arrange part-time status at the place I was at and I started to go to law school for one semester. I took Contracts and Torts. By the time I started to register for my next set of classes, I decided that I really didn't like law. I didn't like the people, I hated the course work, I didn't like going to work during the day and taking classes at night. The schedule was just too much for me. I knew I couldn't quit my job because we had to continue paying for the tuition for both of us, or at least for my husband. I ended up changing jobs to further my career in engineering. I started working for Philips North America.   I started working March 18, 1991, for Advanced Transformer Company in Rosemont, Illinois. My position there was Materials Engineer. The work primarily included trouble shooting production problems and product failure. If raw materials came into one of the plants that was out of spec and we couldn't afford to shut the line down, I had to figure out a way to make it work or I had to make the decision to shut the line down, send the materi-

al back and get the supplier to send us materials that were definitely within spec. I also worked on developing new materials for
newer products or to improve the performance for existing products. It was challenging work. I felt I had finally found a job that
utilized my training in engineering and I was satisfied for the time
being.

Q.
So then how did you make that decision? To actually go to medical school?

A:
I had been interested in becoming a doctor from as early as I can
remember. I had wanted to be a nurse since my mother was a
nurse. My father always used to tell me, "You don't want to be a
nurse. You want to be the boss. You want to be able to decide
what's going on. You don't want to be the one receiving the orders.
You should be the one giving the orders." That really influenced
me a great deal. My father had a profound effect on my life. So as
I grew, I considered becoming a doctor. I thought the human body
was a marvelous machine able to heal itself if given the chance.
The final decision to go to medical school was a kind of a complicated thing. I really had avoided the move because I knew it
would be very difficult. I had exhausted all other career possibilities. I had decided that staying in engineering would not suit me.
Although I was happy at the time, I knew I would not be content
in another ten years.

Q:
So you decided to change?

A:
I decided to change but the decision to change did not come until
my daughter was born. When I was in labor. I remember laying in
bed and watching what the doctors and nurses were doing. I was
amazed at how much science they actually used. I also liked the
way they handled themselves. During the time that I was in labor,
I felt like there was a point when I was staring at the clock that if I
can make it through this, I can do anything.
     When she was born, I started thinking those feelings had
to have been hormonal fluctuations. I decided I cannot change my
entire life on hormones, but several weeks later, I remember looking at her when she was laying in her little bassinet. I was thinking,

"I never wanted her to feel that she couldn't do anything because she was female or because she was too old or because she didn't have enough money or that it involved too much work or that she was disadvantaged for one reason or another."   I thought about how I could teach her to pursue her dreams and recalled that my parents taught me best by example. If I was running away from my dreams because I was afraid I was not strong enough or capable of the hard work, how could I expect her to believe in herself to follow her dreams? My parents and grandparents did their best to teach me to believe in myself. I could not let them down. It was my responsibility to live my life as I saw fit free of fear and doubt. I felt the responsibility to teach my daughter the same values. I realized becoming a doctor would be difficult but I also knew that no matter how difficult something was, if I set my mind to it, there was nothing living or dead that could stop me.

It was a very difficult decision to make. I walked away from a job. I was making about $50,000 at the time. I made more than my husband. We had just bought a townhouse, so we had taken on a lot of new bills and there I was thinking about cutting our income by more than a half. I remember talking to my husband about my thoughts on medical school. He had just come home from work. I was breastfeeding Katherine who was only 12 days old at the time. When he came in, he was basically dragging his rear end on the floor he was so worn out. It was 8 o'clock at night and I knew I had to talk to him because it was bothering me so much. I said to him, " You know I've always been interested in medicine and I wanted to know if you thought it would be a problem if I at least tried to get into medical school. We can do it one step at a time. I have to take the MCAT, figure out if my classes from undergraduate are adequate, apply to schools, see if they were even interested, interview, see if they wanted me, and then go ahead and see if I can find the funding if I got accepted." I honestly thought that man was going to turn around and say, "Are you crazy?" Instead, he just turned around, tired as anything, and he just said, "If you want to do it, do it."

We figured that it would be two years before I could start classes in medical school it all worked out well. I was busy with work and our new baby so I let things go for a little while. My husband actually got on my back about it. Around Christmas that year, he started asking me if I had registered for the MCAT. Finally, I took the plunge and registered for the exam. I also registered for Stanley Kaplan to review for it. I also called some of the schools I would be applying to, to determine if my undergraduate classes were acceptable, if they would be applicable for the biology, chemistry and inorganic chemistry and physics requirements. I had not taken those discrete courses since my discipline had been engineering. I had taken physics ... I had a lot of physics. I had the equivalent of 18 classes in physics. I had inorganic chemistry but I didn't have inorganic chemistry per se. I had chemistry of the solid state, eight thermodynamic classes, polymer chemistry and a host of other classes I cannot remember anymore. I did not know if I knew what I needed to take the MCAT or start medical school.

So I ended up talking to a college advisor at Roosevelt University by the name of Dr. Green. I do not remember how I found out about him, but he was very helpful. I called him to find out what I would need to take to be eligible to apply to medical school because I had not had biology in college. I had not had a formal organic chemistry class in college. After talking to him, he told me, "What do you have to lose? Register for the MCAT, take one of those preparation courses and see if you can score well." I ran through the whole gamut of concerns any student would have: What if I have to take the MCAT twice? And he says, "So you take it twice. If you have a significant improvement in scores, who cares what your first one is?" So I decided to go ahead. Even though I didn't know him, I kind of trusted him. I took the MCAT in April 1993. When my score arrived, I was so nervous I could not open the envelope. Again, my husband came to the rescue and we discovered that I had scored well.

Q:
Without any biology?

A:
No biology in college.   I did have an AP biology course in high school. So I ended up calling my high school biology teacher and asking her about it — was it really considered an AP class? How can I find out — do you have books that I could review?   So I called around and I found out that most medical schools would accept my AP credit if I took an equivalency test. I would just have to prove to them that I knew what was necessary. I ended up tak-ing the test that showed I would have passed the class if I had taken it. Not every medical school required this .. Northwestern accept-ed a letter from my high school biology teacher attesting to the fact that I had done well in the AP class.

Q:

Which schools did you apply to?

A:

I applied to the six schools in the Chicago area which were Chicago Med, Northwestern, University of Chicago, University of Illinois at Chicago, Loyola and Rush, and they all sent me supplementary applications.

Q:

Tell me about your secondary applications.

A:

At this point, it was the kind of thing where they wanted them back in 2 weeks. By then I felt like the pressure was on. I had a lot of things going on at work, but I really wanted to do this. I tried to get my supplementary applications in as quickly as possible to see if anybody was interested in interviewing me. So I did that.

Q:

How did you select your recommendations?

A:

I had my advisor from undergraduate engineering write me a letter of recommendation. He was the academic recommendation. I called the schools and told them that I'm non-traditional — I've been working for 4 years and to ask all my professors to write me letters would be pretty out of date. It's not who I am now. So they said, get your supervisor to write a letter. I knew it would be unwise to ask my supervisor to write a letter. Most people know that it's employment suicide to even let them even remotely know that you would be interested in going into something different.

So there were a couple of people I had worked with and I was currently working with who I knew I could trust. The person I worked with knew I had started law school and thought I had stopped because I had a baby. He sensed I was itching to return to school and just came out and told me if I need a letter of recommendation for law school, I should just let him know. And I said, "Well, okay, law school's one thing, but what about med school?" He was surprised but thought it was a great idea and told me he thought I would make a great doctor. So I explained to him what I needed. Although he was not a direct supervisor, I worked with him on several occasions and he was a manager. He wrote a beautiful letter for me.

Additionally, I ended up going to a man who had a lot of respect for my work . He was Vice President of the engineering division I was in. After contemplating it, I finally ended up sitting down with him and explaining that I felt I had gone as far in engineering as I was going to go within this company. I explained to him off site that I really liked working there, I really liked the work that I was doing, but I knew I would not be content with that in 10 years. At the risk of thinking I'd be the first one on the layoff list, I explained to him that I really wanted to go to medical school. I told him I had already taken the MCAT, scored well and I had started returning the supplementary applications.

He agreed to keep the whole thing in strict confidence and he did the whole time I was there. He wrote me a recommendation because he told me that I had been a very good engineer. He realized that I was serious about going to medical school and fortunately for me, did not take my choice as a personal affront as my direct supervisor later did.

Q

Tell me more about your advisement during the process of applying to medical school.

A:

I went to my doctor to ask him about different schools that were good, and he was a great help. He very candidly told me what he thought of the different schools in the Chicago area. What he had told me was that there was virtually no difference, as far as he could see, among Northwestern, Loyola, Rush-Presbyterian-St. Luke's and University of Chicago. He told me that University of Illinois at Chicago was a school that he knew for a fact accepted more people in the first year than they could afford to keep, and they wanted to flunk them out. He advised me against going there because I was the first one to realize that I would be at a little bit of disadvantage the first year because I had not been into the school swing of things. I was kind of afraid of what to expect because I really didn't know how to study anymore. I didn't even know anybody in school anymore. The people that I had gone to school with who had already gone to medical school were already in their residency by the time I was applying. Any information from them would be old.

My doctor had also told me that Chicago Medical School was a good school to go to if I didn't get in anywhere else because to go to medical school, an accredited medical school, was better than not going to one at all. But he had advised me that if I got into one of the other medical schools, to go there since Chicago Med being a fairly new school, did not have a very established reputation yet.

Q:
Was there anyone else who advised you?

A:
I had gone to my parents. They were always supportive of what I chose to do. My mother, being a nurse, knew what doctors went through and she didn't want my family to suffer. Her biggest concern at the time was, "You're going to stop having babies!" Family is important to all of us since the children are the future. I promised her that my fertility would not suffer solely because of medical school. Although they were reticent initially, they were and are supportive.

I had a friend from Haiti. He told me about his brother-in-law who had gone back to medical school after raising a family. He too had had a totally different career — I think he had been in engineering.   My friend told me, "You have to live your life, whether you're in school or whether you're working, it's going to be hard to have kids. Whether you're in school or working, it's going to be hard to be married, it's going to be hard to have a family, it's going to be hard to have a life. But as long as you fulfill at least a section of each — you have a professional life, educational life, family life, love life, social life — you'll be happy." He gave me a lot of encouragement as far as to go ahead and pursue the dream. Don't let the fact that I was older stop me. Don't let the fact that I had a family stop me. And if I ended up having another baby while I was in school, have it. Be happy, take a little time off. It's not the end of the world.

I think one of the problems that I had to battle personally was that I had it in my mind that there was only one way to go to school. You finish high school, you went to college. You finish college, you went to medical school. I did not realize that you don't have to finish in a certain set of time. That was something that I had learned from my husband by example. He's a engineer. It took him on and off 10 years of going to school part-time and working full-time to complete the requirements for his degree. It doesn't mean he's a worse engineer or a better engineer than someone who finished in 4 years. Maybe by the time he retires, he isn't going to be working as long as a traditional engineer, but who cares? He is doing what he wants to do.

Another issue was age. It bothered me that by the time I finished school, I would be 31 years old. My husband reminded me that he was 32 when he earned his bachelor's degree. He also reminded me that whether I go to medical school or not, I would still be 31 years old some day. I could be 31 and be a doctor or be 31 and not be a doctor .. which did I prefer?

Q:
That's good advice.

A:
So I was fortunate with having a lot of support. I would not be doing this if I did not have the encouragement and the support of my family and friends. That means a lot to me. I hope it means a lot to my kids one day, especially my daughter. As an aside, however, my husband has made sure anyone who was in our lives at the start of this adventure who did not have any encouraging words for this endeavor is no longer a part of our lives. I benefit from his experience in engineering. He knew a few people who did not support his pursuit of his bachelor's degree and he eliminated them from his life when he realized they did not make a difficult task any easier.

Q:
As far as extracurricular activities, obviously you were busy. But were there medically-related activities that you participated in before you went to medical school?

A:
Yes. A lot of my extracurricular activities came from my investigation into how to pay for medical school. I knew that Northwestern made the guarantee that if you were accepted there, they would help you find the money to go, whether it was recommended loans or optional loans, they would help you to find the money to go. I liked that guarantee. But the other schools didn't make the same guarantee but there was no guarantee that I was going to get into Northwestern.

I tried to approach it realistically. Northwestern was my first choice. That's the school I wanted to go to if I was accepted. But I was not as idealistic as I had been when I was younger. I looked into the National Health Service Corps scholarships and I looked into the Illinois Department of Public Health scholarships.

Also the Air Force, Army, Navy. I looked at what it would be like to pay that money back. Even on the anticipated increase of a physician's salary I feared I would not be paying this loan off until I was 80 years old.

I ended up calling the National Health Service Corps and found out that they were very reluctant to give a 1st year medical student such a scholarship. They felt like they were in no position to decide that they wanted to go into primary care.

So I called a gentleman down in Springfield who was in charge of the Illinois Department of Public Health scholarship, talked to him. I basically asked him what I needed to do to qualify for such a scholarship my first year.   I found out all the requirements which were that you had to commit yourself before you entered school to primary care. You could go into internal medicine, general pediatrics, general OB/Gyn or Family Practice. This man down in Springfield, told me that it would be a good idea if I spent some of my free time with some doctors who were in primary care to see if this is what I wanted to do. So I made arrangements to spend time with my OB. Although I had already gone through the experience, I wanted to go through it in a less involved manner. So I spent some time with him, I spent time with the doctor of family practice who cared for my daughter while she was getting her well-baby care. Through him, I also made connections with another doctor of family practice who was a lady who had gone to Northwestern. I also spent time with another doctor who was a doctor of internal medicine. That's how I spent time after work, vacation time and Saturdays for I'd say at least 6 months.   It was really using that experience to decide, is this really what I want to do?   I also spent some time watching surgeons, watching specialists to make sure that I didn't want to do that. And so I was able to decide that yes, I wanted to go into primary care. Exactly which one, I wasn't positive, but I was 95% sure that it was either going to be family practice or OB. So that's how I made that decision. I went ahead and applied for the scholarship. I had to do a lot of writing, calling, interviewing in order for them to accept me into that program.

The Army/Navy/Air Force were out of the picture because my husband said, "I'm willing to follow you around, but not in the Service." We talked about everything. Our lives were consumed with this whole process for probably at least 18 months.

I had learned Spanish in high school. I used it a lot when I was going to South America and Mexico for my job. I did say that I'm semi-fluent. I can have a conversation. I can even talk on the phone in Spanish. And to me, talking on the phone is the hardest thing when you're speaking another language. I did that.

And this whole time, I was also raising my daughter. We've had our blips, but I've had au pairs since Katherine was 12 days old because my boss called me back to work right away.

I can safely say now that I am so glad I made the decision because I am a lot more content. I am mentally more stimulated by what we do. I can see that this profession suits me like a glove while engineering was Okay, but it wasn't a fit like a glove.

Q:
You talked a little bit about your MCAT before and how that helped you with your decision. When did you take it?

A:
In April 1993.   My daughter was still breastfeeding. I guess the administrators of the MCAT are not used to dealing with women who are breastfeeding. I guess this is not a common thing. And I had inquired about being express milk during the test.   And I was told that if I left and turned the test in, I couldn't have it back. I was just there and I tried to hand-express milk. I was very uncomfort- able ard it hurt.

Q:
How did you study for the MCAT?

A:
I ended up taking that Stanley Kaplan review course and that helped me a lot. I went to those classes after work and I also stud- ied at lunch time. I spent a lot of time studying at lunch time when I was at work from those books.   I really liked it. I think if it was- n't for that review course, I would not have scored as well on the MCAT as I did. There were a lot of things that I'd forgotten. I took the MCAT in April because I wanted to apply early. So I thought, maybe it's in my best interest to take the test in April then I don't have to worry about how much time it takes for the score to get in.

Q:
So how long did you study for it?

A:
I registered for the class in December. I got the stuff so I could kind of spend the Christmas holiday reading over it, but the review

course started at the end of January or February. I didn't really get into studying for it until March.

I went to the Kaplan classes, I paid attention, but I started getting antsy the beginning of March because I saw that the time was ticking away. So started spending 3 nights a week after work studying and at least one day during the weekend at Kaplan taking those practice tests. And then I remember taking the virtual MCAT that they offer and I only scored a 40% on that and I was ready to throw in the towel. I really poured on the steam. I figured I don't care how much you suffer, you'll be done on April 17th. So I just put my heart and soul in it, and fortunately I did well enough to get in. I looked at those exams — I mean it's a shame we have to be evaluated on scores and stuff — but if you want to play the game, you have follow the rules.

Q:
Tell me about the day of the MCAT.

A:
I was trying to decide if I should take the day before the test off of work, do I want to run the risk of having them send me out of town on Friday and be gone that weekend and so I took a day of vacation the day before MCAT. I didn't study anything, went shopping, enjoyed my little girl, went home, got a good night's sleep, took the MCAT and that was it.

Q:
That's good. In regards to the AMCAS application, there is a part of it that is non-essay where you list activities and things like that. How did you choose what to include and what not to include?

A:
Well, I did not include any of the employment blurbs. If I didn't work at a company more than a year, I just didn't list them. So I only had two companies on there that I had listed. I focused on the last company I was at because out of the five years I was working, almost 4 years were there. I also tried to avoid putting any gender specific activities. I did not put on the application I was a member of the Society of Women Engineers. I didn't know how something like that would be received. But I did put on that I was a member of the Material Society.   I was an active member of the Metallurgical Society. And the Society of Chemical Engineers.   I tried to stay away from stuff, you know, the garbage you get in the

mail that if you pay x amount of money you're a member of it.

Q:
Tell me about your AMCAS essay.

A:
I remember spending a lot of time on that essay for the AMCAS application.   I made sure that I mentioned the fact that I was married and the fact that I had a family. I talked about the fact that I was an engineer, that was good. So I focused on that. I didn't focus so much on school. I mentioned that I had done research in school and I had done well in school. But that was only 2 lines because it was so long before. Five years before. I focused on the work I did, the responsibilities I had, the fact that I was on call for the plants.

One of things that I tell people when they ask me what advice that you have, I say don't point out anything negative. If you are obligated to point out a negative, turn it into a positive. I mentioned that I had a family. I was able to work it into the essay. It took me a week to write this thing. You write it, you put it on the side, you read it, you revise it. I jammed a lot of information into it.

I never said I was dissatisfied with engineering, and it's the truth. I was happy with engineering, but it just wasn't enough. I was looking for something more, I was looking for more of a challenge. I wanted to use my brain more. I wanted to be able to feel as if I made a difference.

Q:
You were talking about your essay.

A:
I tried to work in as much as I could. My rules of thumb were don't put anything negative in there.   I wanted to try and avoid letting them know that I was female but there was no way of doing that when I said I gave birth. I think that was because of a knee-jerk reaction from some of the discrimination that I had experienced with work. I would always try to put myself in the interviewer's shoes, the reader's shoes. What would I think if this is all I had and I didn't know this person. Would I want to know more about this person? I revised that essay I don't know how many times and the same thing was true with the supplementary applications.

Q:
Tell me about your supplementary applications.

A:
You know with the supplementary applications there were times when they said point out your weakness. I don't want to tell them what's wrong with me. I know what's wrong with me but it isn't anybody else's business. If I was going to write about a weakness, I wanted to think of something that I could turn around and make it a positive. Some of the things that I used were like I was dissatisfied with my knowledge in medicine and I had to do something about this. I had a couple of friends who would proofread for me like my friend, Janis, a coworker. She helped me with my essays. I talked about the business trips I went on. How I was in charge of projects. How I took responsibility for things. How I follow things through to the end.

The secondary applications... I went over those with a fine-tooth comb and some of the people that read my responses would point out the negative and the positive. To turn your weakness into a positive and I think that is an important thing. Don't point out anything negative about yourself. If you're afraid of being too good to be true, well you have to keep in mind that many people don't know you. You have to sell yourself. If you have weaknesses, fine. You know your weaknesses. Don't advertise. Because when you go for an interview they'll figure out what's wrong with you. I mean, my policy has always been don't let people know where your Achilles Heel is because there are those who are going to find it and you don't want to make it easy for them.

I wrote my supplementary essays so that I would have a little bit of a mystique about me. I wanted to give them information about me but I didn't want to tell them the whole story because I wanted whoever was reading to think about me and say, "Oh, I'd love to meet that person." Or leave them with a couple of unanswered questions, giving them just enough information to make it seem like they really want to find out more. Like I guess I would mention about being married or having my daughter has enriched my life so much. Well, how? I would mention it but not explain everything.

I would point out it has helped me to grow in certain ways. But the question would be, "How?" How would that benefit me as a physician. It's like you kind of create the question in their head. How? Why? Why do you think this? How does this work? Or I would say it had a major impact on my life. Can you explain that?

You know, the funny thing was that when I did go for interviews I got those kind of questions. I had already thought out my answers well in advance.

Q:
Tell me about your interviews.

A:
I remember the Northwestern interview was probably the strangest one I went to because it was that panel of three. I remember I went in with one guy who is in my class and another fellow, I can't even remember who he was, but I was totally blown away by those two. I remember thinking, "Oh, my gosh." They're both doctor's kids. They're both fresh out of school. They know how to study. They know this. They know that. And the other guy that was accepted, his name was Paul, at lunch time the two of us sat together and spent the time convincing the other that he would be accepted. You know, you did this research at Johns Hopkins. You did this. You did that. And I remember him telling me, "Yeah, but you've got a family, you've got a kid, you've lived your life. (Not quite I hope!) You know what's going on in the world. You know what it's like to deal with health care.. " We were convincing each other that the other one was going to get in and the funny thing was we both did.

One of the people in the interview asked me... he said something to me about, "Oh, I know why you want to leave engineering. You're doing it for the money, aren't you?" I told him that if I need to make money I can stay in engineering and make enough money to satisfy myself. I am looking for gratification and fulfillment that you cannot buy. I said the fact that you can make money as a doctor is good because I'm going to incur about $200,000 in debt and on top of it I'm going to have to send my kids to school, take care of my husband's retirement, and pay for general living expenses. I don't think I'm going to be living high off the hog.

Before the interviews, even when I was writing the essays, I often though what would these people be asking me. What are they going to be wondering about. They're going to be wondering why I want to leave engineering. They would ask me "do you understand that you're not going to see your little girl grow up. You're not going to be with her every step of the way." Well, if I wasn't going to medical school I would be working and I wasn't with her every step of the way anyway. And to be quite frank, during the last two years in medical school, I spent more time with my daughter than I would have if I'd been working.

Another question that was asked of me was to give him one good reason why Northwestern Medical School should accept me. I told him, well, I really want to be a doctor and I've made up my mind I'm going to be a doctor and I really want to go to the Northwestern Medical School because of the excellent reputation. I told the interviewer, " You'll be saving us both a lot of time and money because if you don't accept me this year I'll just be right here again next year and it's going to cost me money to apply and it's going to cost you money to interview and instead you can just accept me now and by this time next year I'll be towards the beginning of my first year of medical school and we won't have to see each other until graduation." Later, I remember going down the hallway and thinking, " Did I say that? I mean, I don't think I said anything offensive. He was kind of amused. I could see the look on his face and it's like, well. I thought oh, geez. Could I take that back? Did I goof?" But it worked out. I got in. I was in absolute tears of joy I was so happy.

Q:
Do you remember any other specific questions from your interviews?

A:
The biggest ones were why did you want to leave engineering. My response to that was that I did not look at it as leaving engineering. I looked at it as changing materials. I explained to them what I did with my job was I solved problems. I tried to figure out where something went wrong. And that's exactly what you do in medicine. Healthy people don't come to you and say fix my arteries, fix my liver, etc. They're coming to you with a problem or they're coming to you in order to avoid a problem in the future and that's exactly what I was doing as an engineer. And I loved that part of it.

Q:
Did you send extra information to update your application?

A:
Yes. One of the things that I did was my friend, Janice, ended up writing a personal letter of recommendation. I felt it provided information that would be useful to the selection committee yet would

be inappropriate if included in an academic or professional letter.

Q:
How did you decide which school to go to?

A:
You know, my decision of what school to go to had to do with geography, ability to commute, whether or not they had a good attrition rate, paying for it. Prestige entered the equation a little, too. I wanted to go to a school that had a good reputation because something that I also learned when I was in engineering is a year out of school how many As and Bs I had made no difference. It was the name of the school I got my degree from that made a difference. I mean, I worked very hard when I was there and I graduated with a 3.2 cumulative and a 3.8 in my major. I could have so much more fun and still been able to get a job after graduation. (Laughter)   I know I spend less time studying now because I have to take care of my daughter and I have give some time to my husband, and I have extended family.

Q
If you were to give a synopsis of advice to somebody that has some similarity to your situation, what different things that you did would you do differently or what things do you think you did well?

A:
I think the way I handled applying was good. I thought about everything deliberately. I did everything early... as early as I could. I mean, when the AAMC starting accepting applications, it was in the mail in that morning. It was postmarked that day and I called to make sure it was there. I followed up on every little detail. I called people who were writing letters of recommendation for me to the point that .... oh, and the other thing, I read every letter that was sent.   I sealed them and put them in the envelope, along with the business card, and I mailed them. I wanted to make sure that if I was not going to go to medical school it was because the school didn't think I was qualified or I didn't want to go, not because of a third party. I believe in the "Trust but verify rule" made famous by Reagan. I took great care to make sure that people at work did not know that I was applying even though I typed things up while I was there. I took great care during the whole 18 months that I was mulling over this idea, taking the exam, and applying, and interviewing, that they did not know. And they did not know except for

the three who wrote letters for me.

Q:
How about the challenges of having a family while going through medical school and beyond?

A:
Oh, yeah. That was something they questioned me about. I was asked many times if I will be able to handle a husband. Many asked' "Don't you think you're going to have a divorce by the time you're through with school?" I told them that, you know, I'm committed to my husband and I could get a divorce now. I could get a divorce in ten years. I could get a divorce because my job is demanding. I just kept pointing out the fact that I felt school was demanding but that you don't understand how demanding my job is. And, I don't see a whole heck of a lot of difference except the fact that instead of dealing with asphalt plastic, I'm going to be dealing with flesh and blood.

Q:
Any other advice?

A:
Yes. If you're working, don't let your supervisor know even if you have a good working relationship with them. Don't be fooled. If you're doing a good job for them and they like you, they're not going to want to retrain somebody. Don't let them know until you know until two weeks before you leave even though you may know 9 months in advance. When the information gets out, there is no way to take it back. And that was probably one of the most difficult things for me because, when you're excited about it, you want to share it.

Also, don't say anything negative about yourself during the interviewing process even if they ask for it. Anticipate what questions that will come up in an interview about your personal situation. You know, why don't you want to be an accountant anymore? Why don't you want to be an engineer anymore? From my vantage point, stay away from the negative stuff. It's not good to say, "Oh, I'm tired of being an engineer." Because they're going to say how long will it be before you're tired of being a doctor? Point out the positives of what you have to bring to medicine, what you have to offer the school as far as their reputation is concerned.

Whenever somebody tried to point out a weakness, I did

my best, in a few words, to point out to them that they were actually pointing out positives. That was going to be a strength. You have to anticipate because you can't think on your feet about stuff like that. You've got to anticipate it and that's probably the most stressful thing for me because with the essays and the secondary applications, or the supplementary applications, you have time to write, put it off the side, read it, and write again. With an interview you get one chance at each answer so you have to try to anticipate what they're going to ask.

Talk to people who have been interviewed at particular medical schools. See what they're looking for. See what they're asking. Call the Dean.   Call the Admissions Office. They were a good source of information. What are they looking for? What do you look for in an applicant? What is required?

The other thing that I also stayed away from is, granted I'm not that old, but I never mentioned how old I was. I tried not to put dates. I think I was pretty good about never putting any dates. I also never put anything down that would indicate what my race was. I'm conscious of the fact that I've have lost out on opportunities because I'm Caucasian and that irritates me. So on the application even on the areas when it says optional, I would leave the race and gender questions blank. Let them guess. I don't know how sensitive people are but I also pointed out if like I thought it was to my advantage, the fact that I was female. I didn't know if that was too much of an advantage, but I couldn't avoid saying that I gave birth and men don't do that.

Another thing... Somebody asks you an illegal question or a question that is considered illegal. The best way to slit your throat is to tell them, "That it is an illegal question. Or that is an inappropriate question." Answer it, but answer it in a very cryptic way so that they don't get an answer, you know. You answer it but they don't get an answer. I remember when I interviewed up at the Chicago Medical School one of the guys that I interviewed with said to me that I, something to the effect that I must be ancient because I was already married and I had a child and stuff, I had to be so old. And, I think he was just baiting me to try and figure out my age and I said something like , "Age is a matter of mind. If you don't mind, it doesn't matter. It doesn't bother me. Does it bother you?" I said, "You know it's better to get old and die, and what difference does it make if you reach 80, you know, when you're 60 you still have 20 years to go and you know you could be 50 and die at 60 and you only have 10 years to go so whose shoes would you rather be in?" It answers the question but it doesn't give them the information. If you don't want to give somebody information, you don't have to, but you have to anticipate that kind of thing. I think that's probably the biggest challenge in an interview.

I actually had a running list of stuff that I spent six months asking my aunt, my uncle, my husband, my friends, what do you think are potential questions? What would you ask me if you were interviewing me?   I'd say that most of the questions were things that other people had thought of, and I already had my answers ready and so I think I was probably better prepared for applying and interviewing for medical school than I had been prepared for anything else in my life.   I took that as an indication that Divine Providence wanted me to go in this direction.

That's another thing. I had extra-curricular activities as far as my being in church choir and being a eucharistic minister. They have dropped to the wayside. I'm not that active in them now. But, they were definitely pluses on my application.

Q:
Yes, I would think so.

A:
Because it shows that I was in industry. I worked. I volunteered at church. I had a family. I was a big sister for poor kids. My experience as an engineer such as, you know, when I had to go in at 2 o'clock in the morning to take care of an engineering emergency. It indicated that I was on call at weird hours. That I was available. That I responded, you know, these are things that doctors are going to do.

I had no problem with it. It didn't bother me. I enjoyed it. The things that I did was mention that I always took time with my husband. We don't need to go on fancy vacations. We don't have to do exotic things. We're just happy to sit at home and watch a movie or go for a walk or go to the park or take our daughter to the zoo, something like that. I had the undertone that we led a simple life which we do without telling them point blank.

That's probably one of the most difficult things for anybody to do and something that I also did was I asked my closest friends how would they describe me. I remember one application that had a list of words and you had to pick like five of them that described you and write an essay on why they described you. And I just photocopied that sheet a couple of times and gave it to people. I asked them to circle what they thought, what they would describe and why. I just compiled that. I took the stuff that I thought was the best.

Q:
Great idea.

A:
This was a group effort. It still is a group effort. When I say to my husband, "We are going to be graduating in '98" or sometimes I say "We are in medical school." I mean it. I can't do it without my husband. My friends are patient when they do not hear a word from me in six months. My parents are now very supportive. I think they were more reticent about the sacrifices I'd be making because they did not want to see me have a hard life. But, I don't know. It may be a hard life, but I'm a lot happier that I was before. It may be more work, it may be more effort, it may be less sleep but I'm happier. Therefore, the total work output is less.

Q:
Thanks Therese.

Interview Two - Howard Horne

HOWARD HORNE: Howard is forty-one years old and married. He spent the majority of his career working for the New York City Emergency Medical Services culminating as the Associate Director of Service. Additionally, he has worked as a consultant in public health and asset management. Howard received his undergraduate degree as well as a Master of Public Health from the University of Pennsylvania.

Q:
What did you do before you came to medical school?

A:
The majority of my career I was with the New York City Emergency Medical Services in a number of divisions, including Director of Technical Services and Associate Director of the Service. After that I did some public health and asset management consulting while I was taking prerequisites to go back to medical school.

Q:
When and how did you make your decision to go back to school?

A:
 It was a slow decision in coming although I always sort of knew it was going to happen. And I decided I just couldn't deal with my career as it was. I got into the consulting business with the idea of perhaps going back to medical school. This motivated me to get off my behind and take the first prerequisites. General chemistry was one of the classes I needed. When I got an A in general chemistry, I decided I could probably do this.

Q:
What did you originally major in during college?

A:
My undergrad degree was an independent major that is entitled Health Care Delivery and Administration.

Q:
So you obviously had to take additional prerequisite courses. And how did you go about doing that?

A:

O.K. I was living and working in New Jersey just across the George Washington Bridge from New York where a number of legitimate schools exist. There was a small private college in Bergen County which is an affluent county that I thought enjoyed a reasonably decent local reputation and would be adequate to take the post-bacc. courses at. Given that it was a guaranteed ten-minute ride from my office, I could pop in and out and take classes sort of at will whereas going to New York always had the unknown bridge traffic which could be 20 minutes to Columbia or it could mean 2 hours to Columbia and I didn't think that risk was particularly worthwhile, at least in the beginning. As a result, I enrolled in this chemistry class at this small college called Farleigh-Dickinson . I found the quality of teaching having gone to Penn as an under-graduate to be really pretty good. What I didn't quite realize was how bad the advisement situation was, but, also how poor the rep-utation of Farleigh was and how getting an A at Farleigh almost was seen by some Admissions Officers particularly in the area locally to New Jersey as a negative because they said well, just because you can get an A at Farleigh doesn't mean anything and you probably went there because you knew you could get an easy A.

Indeed, also, I think probably the hardest A I'd ever gotten in my life was the A that I got in micro-biology which I took in the summer when I also took organic and was also working full time, that was the summer that I met the woman who was to become my wife. The guy who was teaching it walked in and said, "I'm Dr. Such-and-Such. I didn't get into med school and I know you peo-ple are all here because you want to be. Well, look at me. I'm the St. Peter of med schools." He gave one A. Somehow I got that A. My straight A average at Farleigh didn't mean much.

As a result after an unsuccessful bout in applying, unsuc-cessful for a couple of reasons, I took a physiology class at Rutgers. I also took micro-biology because I needed two biology courses and some schools wanted things more recent than 20 years prior and so I figured I'd need something in the biological sciences that I hadn't taken before and I'd previously taken general bio so I took a comparative physiology course at Farleigh and a micro-biology at Farleigh. And then I took this med school physiology thing at Rutgers.

Q:

Did you have any method in choosing your courses or teachers or did you just choose them because they were offered at a time you could go?

A:
Yeah. There wasn't much selection at Farleigh.

Q:
O.K. In reference to how you studied for your courses, how did you go about that. What materials were the most helpful for you? Lectures, notes, old tests, study groups, tutoring.

A:
I found a study group to be useful in organic. Other than that, I pretty well studied a variety of materials on my own, depending on what the course was. Different courses required different types of effort.

Q:
You said you had some words about the advisement system and your experience.

A:
Another reason to go to a strong school or at least a school where there is some experience in getting people into medical school. Farleigh's advisement service consisted of one 70+ year old physician who also ran their student health service. As a matter of fact, a very unusual circumstance occured during the first year that I applied. I had recommendation packages that were due out and I had requested them early in December. December 22nd came around, Farleigh was closing for Christmas vacation, and I called to see if the packages had gone out and the secretary told me, "No." I said, "What do you mean. They haven't gone out?" She said they haven't gone out. They'll go out after New Year's. I said that's no good. There are schools with deadlines. Nothing I can do. I wrote a motion, presented it to the judge on Christmas Eve day in court. This was the one sitting judge. A Jewish judge who didn't have to go home early for Christmas.

This judge said, "It sounds like they should have gotten those things out. Here's a court order." I went to Farleigh-Dickinson, showed up at the gate, told the security guard that I had a court order to let Professor Jaffee in to mail out my letters and would he call Professor Jaffee and set it up and he laughed at me. The judge had given me on a sheet of yellow paper his home phone. I called the judge on my cellular phone and handed it to the guard. I don't know the exact words that were used. The guard certainly changed his mind fairly quickly. Offered me coffee while we waited for Professor Jaffee. Virtually offered to do everything except shine my shoes. And they got out. But the flip side of that is I went back, in my next go round, I thought I'd circumvent Farleigh and went back to my Alma Mater, Penn, and while they were helpful I found the Penn advisement office tends to play judge and jury a little bit too much. They weren't very encouraging which is probably why I didn't go to med school 20 years ago. The woman who runs the advising office at Penn said to me so what if you had a 3.73 at Penn. I've got twenty one-year olds who have three nines from Penn who aren't getting in so what makes you think you're different. So I ended up using Farleigh the second year.

I figured I didn't need that kind of negativism. But, yeah, but it was pretty much "do it yourself."   I think checking up on your advisement very important.

Q:
Obviously, you have a lot of work experience in the medical area and in the non-medical area. Tell me a little about your medically-related experiences and how you think those helped you to get in.

A:
I guess the biggest help was knowing physicians and knowing physicians at a level to give me the advice that I couldn't get at Farleigh-Dickinson in terms of selecting schools. Since then I have found that physicians are not necessarily the best people to help you select schools. But, in terms of general mentorship, useful. Certainly, when it came to getting letters of recommendation that was useful because most of the people who I knew at Penn were either dead or gone. Certainly, my experiences in medicine are useful in some areas. And I think will be more so as I get into more clinical things because there seems to be a great reticence of many medical students to jump into medical things whereas I've never been accused of being sullen or apathetic when it comes to jumping into clinical situations and I think that comes from experience.

Q:
What other extra-curricular activities were you involved in?

A:
A number of things. Largely professionally related. I was a member of a volunteer ambulance squad. I was on the Board of a community development corporation. I was on the Board of a senior citizens center. I was a Red Cross instructor. At some point given

what I did for a living vocation and avocation sort of mixed.

Q:
Now I'd like to talk about your favorite test and mine, the MCAT. When do you recommend taking the test, spring or fall ?

A:
It's a loaded question. I say fall even though I didn't do that because spring was too late. Fall the previous year. Spring for me I found it to be too late.

Q:
O.K. Excellent. Did you take any review courses?

A:
I started to take a local review class. I didn't get much out of it so I didn't do much with it.

Q:
Then how did you organize your studies?

A:
Practice exams. Any of the ones I might get my claws on. I mean, I must have done fifteen. I did all of the old ones that they published. I did all of the ones that were in any MCAT review book I could find. As I say, I probably did a minimum of 15 practice tests. Because it was not so much learning the material as learning the "bubble jet" head stuff. When I went to Penn and even at Farleigh we did not have multiple choice tests and I'm still not comfortable with multiple choice tests.

Q:
How long did you study for the MCAT? What was your approach?

A:
Some evenings, probably one evening a week from November until January or February and then I started studying more and more on weekends. I was also taking physics at the same time and I was working full time. I took two weeks off to study for the MCAT.

Q:
And the AMCAS essay? And non-essay part? You, obviously, have more than you can fit in the allotted space. Especially in the non-essay part? What was your point that you tried to stress?

A:

The point that I tried to stress was that number one, there was a logical progression toward medicine in what I've done and that the work that I was doing was patient care oriented. I also included a little bit of family history, a little bit of the motivational aspects of why I wanted to do this, and a little bit of discussion about why I felt a returning student would be an asset to the profession.

Q:

Tell me about your AMCAS essay.

A:

My essay. I talked about the circuitous route that I took to getting here, why I interrupted my education, what I'd done that related to undergraduate, the fact that my father and grandfather were physicians. I mean, I had a variety of things to say and that may have been my only chance to present it. I compacted it. I became very good at working with computer fonts. My advice is that everybody buy an IBM Selectric and a printer with a straight paper pack.

Q:

For the secondary applications, how did you use those? What was your general impression? What essay questions stick out in your mind?

A:

I developed the secondary, what I call the base supplemental essay, and tried to fit it into wherever I could. I put everything on the computer. Grab it, modify it, hit it and run. But I had two years to do this so I had to be better at it after the first go round. So I had the secondary material sort of categorized, organized.

Q:

That's great. Did you update your application after the secondaries? Did you send additional information?

A:

The first year I did send additional grades. The second year I think I sent a couple of "suck up" letters to certain schools, when I finished a research project. But the application process the second time around was sort of short. I knew where I thought I wanted to apply early.

Q:
O.K. So do you believe in applying very early?

A:
Let me tell you about the first year and let me tell you about the second year. The first year I got married. Despite my best intentions of getting this stuff out early it didn't necessarily happen. Despite my best intentions I decided to get things in by the deadline. That was a mistake. I got a lot of wait lists and a lot of traveling. And a lot of calling to try to work my way up the wait lists and I didn't get in.

The next year I showed up in Washington at AMCAS on June 14th at 8 a.m. thinking that there would be a line around the block and I had a bet with a physician friend of mine that there would be at least 150 people. At 9 o'clock a security guard came down and ushered us on to the elevator. There were 11 people. I was the 11th on the elevator. Because I was the last one on, I was the first one off and handed my paper across the desk at 9:03 a.m. The thing that upsets me is that I wasn't #1. Somehow 300 applications, 352 actually, got in there before mine and I was number 353.

Nonetheless, I was in there early and I got every supplemental out within three days of its arrival but I'd seen most of these supplemental before from the same schools. Did a little bit of refining and I got myself a better printer so I could get them out quicker.

Q:
O.K. And you think that makes a big difference?

A:
I think that makes a big difference. I mean, I got an interview at what was then my first choice school the first week that this school was interviewing and I heard 2-1/2 weeks after that. Maybe I should have continued applying a little bit harder.

Q:
How did you choose the schools that you applied to?

A:
The first year I sat down with a physician friend of mine who was actually the Medical Director of the largest voluntary hospital in New York State. He and I went through the AMCAS guide book and selected a large number of schools to which I applied based on

criteria I used, he used, some that both of us used, some we agreed on, some we didn't agree on. The next year I sort of did the same thing, but I applied to a few less state schools, out of state, because I thought that was largely a useless proposition.,

A very wise fellow, a fellow down at Tulane said "cast a wide net when you're an older student." And I agree that is the case.

So cast a wide net to a variety of schools of varying difficulty. There's no safety school anymore. Not only is there no safety school, but I have found that if you are an older white male don't waste your time at the bottom half. I say that flippantly because there is no school, no application, worth wasting your time as an older student in today's market.   But it was not until I was accepted at Northwestern, and I believe the other schools know when you're accepted, that I even got an interview with a school that is ranked in the bottom half.

The bottom half schools are looking at numbers, numbers, numbers. And tens on the MCAT aren't good numbers to them. I worked at URWJNJ on a research project a couple of years prior, was the only non-physician on their health care outcomes committee, only non-faculty member on their health care outcomes committee. A member of that committee is also a member of the Admissions Committee and wrote on my recommendation that I was better that 90% of the people he interviewed. That school is only interested in numbers and they want youth and they want diversity and white males with tens, particularly, and even straight As from Farleigh-Dickinson don't count.

Q:
How did you choose your recommendations? You had a big number to draw from.

A:
My premedical program at Farleigh does a composite recommendation which is not good because it doesn't say anything. It's like a boiler plate. So to supplement that, I got Farleigh to agree to send out three non-Farleigh letters which they will send out in their entirety.   I used one from the highest ranking doctor that I could find that I had ever worked with who was a close friend and mentor and who was the Chief Medical Officer at the Emergency Medical Services and was also the Chief Medical Officer at the largest voluntary hospital in New York state. Another one I used was a client who, for me this is hard to say.. an attorney, was corporate counsel for the District of Columbia, and the other was a

close friend who could speak on the personal level and he had also been and is a high ranking government official. So it's more than he is just an attorney. He had been the Chief Budget Officer for the Governor of the State of New Jersey in Washington. Those got included.

 Additionally, one professor who had read my recommendations, who knew me quite well, felt that the Farleigh recommendation was, you should pardon the expression, fairly blasé and, as a result, he took it upon himself to conduct a letter writing campaign on my behalf. I provided him with the labels and he quickly mailed a heck of a lot of letters on my behalf. It didn't hurt that this guy saw me save somebody's life in a restaurant.

Q:
What different types of interviews did you have?

A:
I had students, I had single professors, I had dual professors, I had professors. One school, name won't be mentioned, during a snow storm on the day that they bombed the World Trade Center, we were supposed to have two faculty interviews. Instead we had one. The guy met me, and said I don't usually do this but they got me to do this today. Do you mind if we stop by the men's room and start there because I gotta go. So we started the interview in the men's room. At the end of the interview the guy said you sound like an interesting guy. I'm going to tell them to take you.

I had interviews with students. Some places the students said they had input in the decision making process. I found the interviews by psychiatrists to be the worst. I had some real interesting discussions with some interviewers that I really felt like I enjoyed and everybody learned something. One of those was with a fellow in Syracuse, I believe, the day that Hillary Clinton was going to give her first health care speech. So that was sort of interesting.

Q:
Do you remember any specific questions that the interviewers asked you?

A:
I can remember some I don't like. Including the ones who probably blatantly violated the law by saying I was too old to be applying to medical school. The thing I disliked the most were interviewers who tried to tell me I should pursue other career paths.

Q:
What would be some general recommendations that you'd give to a non-traditional person that was applying to med school?

A:
Apply early, apply to a lot of schools, stress why you want to go to medical school, what you have done in life either recently or over a period of time that applies to medicine, why what you have done will make you a better physician or a physician with some special skill that other people might not have.

Q:
Thanks Howard.

Interview Three - Joanne Zell

JOANNE ZELL: Joanne is twenty-seven. She graduated from Michigan University with a degree in Psychology. After college she worked as a National Parks Ranger at the Grand Canyon and later as a counselor for emotionally disturbed children.

Q:
What did you used to do and tell me something about how you were you motivated toward medicine?

A:
I was a psych major, graduated from Michigan in '91 and I immediately went to Grand Canyon and worked as park ranger for the summer and then, after that, I moved to Boston and I taught environmental education for a month, until it got too cold . Then I moved to Oregon and I worked for a year and a half as a counselor for emotionally disturbed kids. Let's see. During that time, I got an ENT certification and enrolled in classes at Portland State University.

Q:
So how do you make that decision that you wanted to go to medical school?

A:
Well, , I think I was always interested in medicine. I think that I didn't have the confidence to go through the application process when I was younger or even the drive, to be honest. During my undergraduate years , a friend who was a premedical student always said that he was an over achiever and I was an under achiever. And I don't know that that was totally true but I think that I certainly wasn't ready to make any huge career decisions at that time. And I knew that I liked working with people on social issues. I remember when I was graduating I talked to this one woman one day. She said, "Yeah, I'm going to this post bacc. program at Loyola. I'm gonna go to med school." I said, "Gosh, I've always wanted to do that." She said you can. You know, with these programs people do it all the time and she's at Rush now. I don't know. I just kinda kept that in the back of my mind, I always thought that I might go to medical school but it was just a question of when.
When I was in college I thought I might go to social work

grad school. And then it was social work and public health and then I wanted to work in a hospital with patients and I kept sort of choosing these career decisions that were as close to being a physician as possible. Then finally one day I said this is silly. Everything is pointing at one thing and I think I just need to take the risk. I was afraid I wouldn't get in and I was making this huge commitment and both of these things really scared me.

So the getting certified as an ENT, for me, was like a first step. I figured it I liked it. It was just scratching the surface but I figured if I liked it and it came easily to me then I would keep going and that's exactly what happened. I loved ENT.

Q:
So you had no science courses before premed?

A:
No. Except like bio, psychology or something like that, you know, that's the only science class I took at Michigan. I avoided them like the plague otherwise.

Q:
So you had to take premedical classes. Which ones did you take?

A:
While I was still working I took first year chemistry at Portland State. Then I realized this is just too slow, you know.   So   I quit my job and moved back to Chicago and I was going to enroll in Loyola and take the other ones which would be organic, physics, and bio. I enrolled in one of those 9-week Summer physics courses, I means it covers a year of physics - don't do it. I took it at Northwestern and it was a calculus-based physics because I thought that if I could survive calculus-based physics that I could convince any admissions person that I didn't have to take calculus. I had taken it when I was a junior in high school and I didn't want to take it again.

Q:
Did you have a year of it in high school?

A:
Yeah. Actually I had college physics and chemistry in high school as well.

Q:
Did you have credit for that?

A:
I had a year of college credit for the physics. And a half year of calculus.   I had advanced background but it was 8 years before so I
took this physics class and then I enrolled in Loyola and I took bio
and organic together for a year. Then It was done.

Q:
Did you take any advanced courses after that?

A:
 I really took the bare minimum. I was the epitome of bare bones.
And, to be honest, I think people should be required to take more
science. I do. I think it's a huge disadvantage.

Q:
How did you pick your teachers for you premed courses?

A:
Except for maybe second semester at Loyola it was a guess-tima-
tion. I knew the teachers by then and I specifically chose a woman
teacher for biology who is a really good teacher. I heard great
things about her.

Q:
 And what materials did you find most helpful when you were in
the classes? What did you use as your main study aids? How did
you study?

A:
Well, depends on the class, you know. Usually, the actual text
book came out with a study guide you had questions and I did a
lot of that. Like organic, I just would sit and do problems over and
over and over and over again until I understood it.

        Personally, for me, anything that's hard, drawing diagrams,
I do a lot of stuff like that. I mean, I even like it. I love physics
problems. I'm serious. To sit down with a big blank piece of paper
and a juicy physics problem, draw lots of pictures, and, you know,
even if you don't figure it out you've got this great thought process
that you can show to someone and you can say, "Oh, this is why,
where you weren't thinking right."

Q:
Did you use study groups or any tutoring or anything like that?

A:
Yeah. When I was at Portland State they had like a science tutor center and I would go. There was a chem tutor if I had any questions. I always actually go to professors a lot. I find that extremely helpful and also the teacher gets to know who you are which I always think can't hurt. I mean, at Loyola I remember first quarter my teachers told me I was the only person who came to see them. It was just really nice. They have a lot to share and you really get advice and they'll ask you about yourself and then you can also definitely get a recommendation.

Q:
All right.. How about advisement? Did you use any school advisors for either your class schedule or for applying to medical school?

A:
Well, basically, one of the reasons that I moved to Chicago to go to Loyola is because I had heard this was a program specifically for older students and it would include an advisor and I thought that would be great. They did have a center there where they handled all your recommendations for you. You know, you send them all there, and they would send them out, whereas, a lot of older students don't have that kind of access anymore to undergraduate advisement.

So I thought that was really helpful, plus they had people's interviews on file. After I had an interview, they would send you a sheet and you would fill out as many questions as you could remember and they would send it back to Loyola and have them all compiled. So if you have an interview at a specific medical school, you can see and go and see what this person's impression, who did they interview with, and what did this person want to know.

Also, I did call a Dean of Admissions at Northwestern, and talked to her for a while. I think one thing to suggest is to meet people from different schools. A lot of the schools will meet with you. I went on tours. I went to a osteopathic school here in Chicago. I went on other tours last year. If they'll see you go and talk with them.

Q:
Tell me about your extra-curricular activities, both medical and non-medical. What do you think has helped you for your medical school application?

A:
When I was an undergrad, I did everything under the sun. I worked in the psych center, counseled children, tutored as a big sister. I volunteered at the Grand Canyon Clinic during the summer while I was in college. During my post-bacc., I actually didn't have as many extra-curricular activities. I didn't have as much free time, but I volunteered at Children's Memorial Hospital for a year, volunteered at Northwestern Memorial Hospital for half a year. I did it because I felt I needed more exposure. I mean, I worked, I think '93 for the whole summer, I worked as a EMT , so I got a lot of medical experience.

What else? I ran a marathon. I put that on all my applications. I thought that was kinda juicy, you know.

Q:
How about the MCAT? When did you take it? How long before you applied? And, when would you recommend taking it?

A:
I took it April, in the spring. I was applying that summer so I took it in April. I would recommend April because then you can always retake it.

Q:
Did you take a review course?

A:
Yeah. I took Kaplan. I don't know. I'm glad I took it, actually. I felt that it covered some weak points. There definitely were things covered in Kaplan that I realized were on a lot of MCATs that were never covered in some of my classes. Not huge points but little physics things like mirrors, you know, things I didn't learn in physics. I found it really helpful because they had done all this research on what shows up on the MCAT.

Q:
How about stuff from MCATs?

A:
Oh, yeah. I took the old MCAT practice tests. I had so many practice MCAT tests and I used them all. I took test after test after test
for months before MCAT. I would choose a section, take the section as a practice test, and then go through it question by question
with a friend. Then we would start doing more until we did a
whole MCAT practice test at once.

Q:
Well, how long did you study?

A:
I studied for six months. I was really worried. I'm not a great test
taker and I was really concerned. I mean not intently, intently, but
I was in school, too. I studied at night. I had a million books. I
think that Flowers book was pretty good. I thought that was pretty
good.

Q:
O.K. How about your AMCAS application? What did you try to
emphasize? Your post -bacc or your college?

A:
Definitely post -bacc. I really focused a lot on working with emotionally disturbed kids and I really pushed this whole mind/body
connection thing. I've used that a lot. I mean, I gave it to a friend
of mine and he said it's very you but it's a little "touchy-feely" for
med school.

Q:
So what did you write in your essay?

A:
Just something my friend told me. She's at Stanford now, but she
said that most of the applicants need to write how they got to
where they are. It's really a lot easier for us, you know what I'm
saying? We don't have to be cute or anything. Really, you need to
explain what you're doing, you know, and so mine was sort of a
chronological look at how I made my decision. My big push has
always been that I've been dedicated to social service and in the
end the idea is that I'm still really dedicated to that. I just see
myself using a different form to reach the same goal. I used the
mind/body thing more to connect all the work that I did with the
medicine to go from like social work to medicine. My big push

was that I've been a social servant all my life. Period.

Q:
How did you choose the schools that you applied to? Did you apply all over?

A:
I have to say in some ways it was haphazard. I mean I hit certain areas by geography. I applied in Chicago mostly because I thought it would be a little easier for me being from Chicago. Then I chose schools like Portland, San Francisco and Seattle for location.

Q:
What were the most important factors?

A:
Definitely location and then I started to look at Penn which I heard looks favorably at post-bacc. students so I thought I'll give it a shot. I knew it was a really good school. And then the other couple of schools that I applied to out of state I either felt I was sort of look-ing at their stats and I was a good candidate for them like Michigan for example. At Michigan I knew that I actually had a little con-nection there, so I applied there. I just chose Michigan State because their school was more focused on primary care so I had different reasons for almost every school. I wanted to apply to a lot of schools.

Q:
Tell me about your secondary applications.

A:
I think I ended up filling out the secondary for 14 schools. I think it was a really good number. I mean it worked out well for me.

Q:
How about your recommendations?   How did you choose your recommendations?

A:
I had already on file at Michigan something like six or seven rec-ommendations, so, I've always known I wanted to go to grad school so I think that was a plus 'cause I had 2 in my file that I could use. They were very general for character recommendations from col-lege, you know, that long ago. I felt like I had a really nice mix

because I had those and I had two science ones from Loyola and then I had my boss at the psych. hospital. Also, I had one from the doctor that I worked with. He was my boss. I worked his the lab the year I was waiting to get in and I had a letter from him.

Q:
Did you send any additional information or letters?

A:
I really didn't have anything at Michigan other than my father was very involved there.   Personally when it came to undergrad I was very proud I went to Michigan. I still had the same connection but I made my father swear he wouldn't get involved at all. But I think for this endeavor, you know, your ego is nothing, you know, whoever you can talk to help you is good. Oh, and my Dad had a friend who was on the Board at U of C who I went and talked to. I mean, I talked to everybody. Whether they wrote me a letter or not. I talked to anybody who had any connection with any school just for information because it made you a little more informed when people are interviewing you.

Q:
Tell me about your interviews.

A:
Some guy asked me on an interview, how do we know that you're not going to give up on medicine like you gave up on social work? I said, "I don't think I've given up on anything."   You know, he thought he had me.

Q:
Okay, thanks.

Interview Four - Sandeep Dave

SANDEEP DAVE: Sandeep is twenty-seven years old. He received
an undergraduate degree in India and subsequently a Master of
Biomedical Engineering Degree at Northwestern University. Prior
to medical school, he worked as a systems analyst.

Q.
You're 27, so you started when you were 26. What did you do·
before coming to medical school.

A.
I was trained as a computer science major. I was a systems analyst
for two years. I quit my job to get a master's in biomedical engineering. Then after that I started medical school.

Q.
How did you decide to go back to medical school?

A.
It was a fairly long process. There was no one point in time that I
can say that's when I made the decision. It was more of a contin-
uous thing. I quit my job to get a master's in biomedical engineering. I was already moving in that direction.

Q.
At that point, did you know that you wanted to go to med school?

A.
Not really, but once I was in grad school I got more exposure and
we had interaction with people who were MDs and doing some
kind of research. But I saw that they got to do more than just play
with electrodes in a lab all day long. You know, see patients and
that kind of thing. That interested me more. . A year more of
research convinced me that I didn't want to do any research anymore anyway. I got a lot of support along the way from my grad
school advisor, from other MDs, and so on and a lot of people
helped me along the way also.

Q.
 Because you had an engineering background some of your prereqs would have been included, obviously, but did you have all of
them?

A:

No. I didn't have any biology. I had no chemistry. I had enough physics to last me a life time. And I didn't have any English and some schools require that. I never had college level English. I got my biology requirements through the biomedical engineering degree. And, I took biochemistry before taking organic chemistry or anything. And then I took organic chemistry at one of the local schools. English I took at Northeastern Illinois.

Q:

So you did end up taking a year of English.

A:

Two semesters, well, two courses. Which was great because it was like the easiest thing I've ever done except for creative writing which was my other English course, probably harder than bio-chemistry. I got a book of poems out of that. It was a lot of work.

Q:

Did you have any system of choosing the courses or the professors.

A:

My schedule was the thing and cost. I took some courses at a state school to conserve on total cost.

Q:

What different materials did you use to study. What did you find most helpful?

A:

I review old exams and I was in pretty good shape to begin with. I just went over textbooks and I would read like I was reading for pleasure and some things stuck. I studied alone.

Q:

All right.. As far as extra-curricular activities, which medical and non-medical activities did you participate in?

A:

Well, research was not exactly extra-curricular, although I did start off in research at the Rehab Institute while I was still working. When I was in school, I was in the Emergency Room as an orderly at the hospital. That's pretty much it. Most of my stuff was non medical. I used to be an English as a second language instructor,

then later on I was on the Board for three years and so on so I did
a lot with that.

Q:
So as far as the MCAT went, did you take it in the spring or the fall?

A:
Well, actually, I took them twice. I took them in the spring and I
didn't do as well as I thought I would and then I retook them in the
fall.

Q:
How did you study for the MCAT?

A:
I never studied for the MCATs, per se. There was always something
going on and I had to present a paper right before the MCAT so I
didn't study for the MCATs the way a lot of people do. The only
thing I did to prepare for the MCAT was to do the old MCAT exam.

Q:
And the AMCAS application? For the non-essay part, where you
put your activities, what did you try to include?

A:
I mean some things shouldn't be there. You write an article for
some school magazine, that's ridiculous if you include that in an
application. I was captain of the Debate team and that kinda
belongs there. I got an award for my undergraduate research project and that was there. Things like that. I mean, once you have a
list, you know how much space you have and you can kind of, you
know, play with that.

Q:
For your essay what did you write about?

A.:
It was an autobiography. It was my life story in kind of a medical
way, talking more about my decision to go to medical school and
so on.

Q:
Tell me about your secondary applications. I'm sure you filled out
a few of those. Do you remember any general impression or spe-

cific questions that stick out in your mind?

A:
I had the AMCAS essay so I could pretty much tailor that to the secondary applications.

Q:
Did you send extra materials?

A:
All the time. I had a couple of publications happen during that year so when they were about to happen I would let them know and when they did happen I would let them know. I would call them all the time and send letters. Actually a couple of the schools asked me to stop sending them stuff.

Q:
Really. Do you think that helped you?

A:
It couldn't have hurt. It may have helped. Most schools will simply not respond, as you probably know. They won't reject you and they won't ask you out for an interview either. So those are the schools you need to work on.

Q:
Right. Do you think timing is important?

A:
Oh, absolutely. Apply as early as you can.

Q:
And how many schools did you apply to?

A:
Twenty-seven.

Q:
How did you choose those?

A:
I pretty much chose every school that would accept someone who went to a foreign undergrad program. A lot of schools have explicit policies against foreign undergrad schools. For example,

Northwestern does. And some schools have humanities requirements and so on and often times I didn't meet those. Some schools
are very heavily in state and there's no point in applying to those.
So any school that took a significant, and by significant I mean
20%-30% maybe, number of out of staters and did not require a US
undergrad degree I applied for.

Q:
And your recommendations. Obviously, you would have a large
number of people to ask. How did you choose the people you did
ask to write recommendations for you?

A:
I chose on the basis of popularity with the medical field. I didn't
want someone that was talking on and on and on about things that
may or may not be relevant. That was good because I was in a biomedical engineering program where everyone was in medicine or,
actually worked with someone who was. That worked out very
well. A Chairman of a Department for one. My research advisor,
of course. Mostly academic. I would give the people writing recommendations my AMCAS essay so they knew more about me than
just the contact we've had.

Q:
 And your interviews. What were the different styles?

A:
Mostly they were one on one. Usually they were multiple so you'd
have one interview and then a second interview. Sometimes the
second would be with a student. Sometimes it was just one interview. Northwestern, of course, was a panel.

Q:
Were there any questions that you remember that were especially
good or especially bad?

A:
They were pretty much run of the mill. Why do you want to be a
doctor? Some of them asked for political stuff, Medicare,
Medicaid, that kind of thing.

Q:
Did they ask you about your background at all?

A:

Oh, absolutely. My AMCAS essay gave them so much material. I guess I like to talk so most interviews were sort of a funny experience for me. Most of the schools I interviewed at I got in.

Once I had an interview, I always thought I was already in. I mean, Northwestern, it was ridiculous. I was rejected once. I was here like laughing and joking and even during the interview I had a hard time keeping a straight face.

Q:

And how did you choose the schools that you wanted to attend?

A:

I wanted to stay in Chicago. The only other school I would attend, if I didn't go here, was probably Stanford. I was accepted by Penn which is much, much higher rated, but I didn't want to go there. I was looking for a pass/ fail system . I was looking to stay in a place I knew and Northwestern I knew really well. Very high on my list.

Q:

Is there any general advice that you'd want to give somebody who was non-traditional, maybe with your background?

A:

Apply early. Build as many bridges as you can as early as possible. I knew the Dean of Admissions at all the schools in this area. I met every one. Call and make an appointment. Sometimes it's hard because they don't like to talk to people but I would tell them I have a really good friend and this and that. For them it helps to have a face when the application does arrive. And Northwestern, they have a great Dean of Admissions. I was rejected in November but he was still giving me advice on how to deal with other schools and so on. It was nice to have someone that supportive.

Q:

Great. Thanks Sandeep.

Interview Five - Margy Aitken

MARGY AITKEN: Margy is twenty-nine years old. She worked as
a professional medical illustrator and creative director for a medical chart company and later ran her own business as a free-lance
medical illustrator. She received her undergraduate and Master of
Medical Illustration Degrees from Michigan University.

Q:
What did you do before you came to medical school?

A:
I was 28 when I started medical school. I was a medical illustrator
before that. I got my undergraduate degree at the University of
Michigan. I got a Master's degree in Fine Arts in medical illustration from the University of Michigan. I took one year off in
between undergrad and graduate school. I moved to Chicago after
graduate school in 1991. I worked for two years as a medical illustrator and creative director for a medical chart company. I quit my
job in order to work free lance for two reasons. One was to see if
I preferred working free lance and would consider staying in the
field of medical illustration. Two, to give me the flexibility of time
in order to go back to school to get the premed classes that I didn't
take before.

Q:
So when did you make your decision to go back to medical school?

A:
It first occurred to me that it was something that I wanted to do
while I was in graduate school finishing my degree. And I was
counseled to finish my degree, get a job, see if I liked it, and then
reevaluate what I wanted to do with myself. So, although I was
thinking about it in 1989, I graduated in '91, I worked until '93, and
even in '93 I still hadn't made the decision to actually do it. So
that was when I started taking classes. I needed three courses. I
had biology. I needed chemistry, physics, and organic . I didn't do
it right. I would not tell anybody to do it the way I did it. I took
night classes and I worked as an illustrator during the day. They
were in Evanston and I was in Chicago so I had a forty-five minute
commute. So I was going to Evanston twice a week at night. They
were 3 hours, each class. And then I had labs on Saturdays. And
I did that for a year. For the school year. And then I made my deci-

sion. After those classes. Because I started those in the fall and then I took MCAT in March. So I had to decide to go through with it.

Q:
And your classes. Did you choose them in any specific manner? Who were the teachers?

A:
I wanted to have the best name I could on my transcript. I knew that Northwestern had a night school and that it was no different on your transcript than the day school and it was cheaper. So I signed up.   And they were really cheap, I mean relatively. Northwestern charges about $2,300 a class and they were $600. So they were really cheap.

But the physics class they had was calculus-based physics and I hadn't had any calculus. So I called the professor and I said, "You know I haven't had any calculus. What do you think?" He said, "No problem." I remember him saying that. No problem. The tests do not require calculus. You'll be fine. Well, sure the tests don't require it but, I'll tell you, for the day to day work you had to have calculus to understand what he was talking about. They did math problems across the board until the cows came home and I had to be able to understand what he was doing. So I learned a lot of calculus and it was great because I had an application for it. I had the physics, the mechanics of physics to learn it which made it easier to learn and I was learning physics at the same time.

So it was actually pretty cool. But I had enough of that after about one semester and I dropped it. And I finished my physics classes at DePaul. DePaul was a lot more expensive. It was about $950 a class a quarter so my $600 a semester went up. That was bad but it was close to my house.

Then I made my biggest error, I think. I took MCAT in March and I hadn't finished physics or chemistry and I hadn't had any organic. Luckily, I was studying at the law library downtown and I met this guy who was a first year law student who had gotten his Ph.D. in biochemistry at Northwestern and had taught for a little while. So, he said Kaplan, you know, takes me on every once in a while to teach their classes. If you want, I can coach you on how to take the test. And I said, "Coach me?" And he said, "Yeah, you haven't had any organic. But you can still answer the questions without knowing any of the material. So he did. So I didn't do as poorly as I could have. I didn't hurt myself but I certainly didn't score well. I wouldn't suggest that.

Q:
O.K. What materials did you use to study in your classes? The text book, problem sets, old tests?

A:
Text books which I think explains why I'm a poor test taker. I read what they told me to read. I did the problem sets in the book. I was a good student. Night school was all older students and, I don't know, I think it was easier for sure.

Q:
Did you study in groups at all?

A:
Yes. I had a couple of good friends. One was a lawyer downtown. The other was a secretary at a law firm. And they were both good to study with.

Q:
As far as advisement goes, did you use any of the advisors from the department?

A:
I came down, at the University college they have a guy who does all the post-bacc advisement. I liked him a lot. Then I came to Northwestern and I talked to the Admissions Office. They basically said don't even bother to apply here because you won't get in. I applied anyway and disregarded them.

Q:
Did you use an advisor for planning your class schedule and for applying specifically? What did you use your advisor for?

A:
Timing my application. I used the university college advisor for timing it. I used him for financial advisement and for which courses to take. I don't think I was the only one in his office looking for that. Although he was just the University college advisor, he knew what I needed and he knew how to get me into it. I ended up taking organic chemistry in the summer, speaking of advisement. I went to Northwestern in Evanston and I spoke to one of the deans up there. So I went and spoke to the Dean and I said, "Listen, you know, this is what I need. I need to take organic this summer. The Dean looked at me and said, "Don't take that class. It is so hard

you'll never get through it." And I thought, I'm a smart girl. I can get through that. That's summer organic. So I took it.

I have never been more miserable in my life. Never. Not even in medical school. That was the worst form of torture I'd ever even talk about. And I could only get through six weeks of it which was two quarters. So it was a nine-week, one-year organic accelerated class. It was bad. I got through two quarters of it and that's all you needed. Somebody whispered to me in the front row, "Hey, you don't need that last quarter of organic. You can take bio-chem instead. And supplant that final quarter. I would suggest that to everybody. Because I don't think you need that much organic.

Q:
Tell me about your extra-curricular activities.

A:
I went into the OR a lot because I was drawing it. I worked in my client's office when he was there so I had a lot of patient contact, , so I had an idea of what goes on. I at least knew what it was like to be in the medical field. It was good.

Q:
How about your non-medical extracurricular activities?

A:
I was in a lot of professional organizations, associations, groups, etc.

Q:
Okay, we talked about your MCAT. You didn't take a review course, but you had a private tutor basically that helped you study for it. And you took it in March?

A:
I wouldn't suggest that. You score higher in August overall. If you can do it, I would take it in August. Exactly. I would take it the year before, the August before the year you apply. If you're going to apply June 15 of 1996, I would take it in August of 1995.

Q:
How long did you study for it and how long would you recommend studying for it?

A:
I bet I studied a month with work. It's hard for me to say what is the ideal amount of time to study. I still think a month is the ideal time. I don't think you can retain very much more than a month before that. I had recently learned the material so it was still pretty fresh, except the biology which I hadn't done in about 8 years. So that was cold, down right chilly. But I don't think it mattered because the biology section wasn't fact recitation anyway. It tested your ability to read and understand laboratory-type work passages and then relate that to problem-solving type thinking. I don't think the MCAT measures your ability to know facts, it measures your ability to solve problems.

Q:
On to the AMCAS. We talked about the non-essay category. What did you include and what impression you wanted to make?

A:
I did work in a lab, but in graduate school in a radiation/oncology lab for a year about 10 hours a week. The guy I worked for was really intimidating. Anyway, so I put that kind of stuff on there. I put what I did for a living. I put some of the awards I won related to my job. I basically wanted them to know I wasn't leaving my career because I wasn't good at it. I was choosing to change jobs. And I thought that was a really important point for me because — I don't know if that would apply to everybody — going into medicine isn't just a default career. I think that's really important.

Q:
Do you remember your essay?

A:
I think I wrote how I was counseled not to go to medical school. It wasn't a real moving story. It was more an explanation. And the things that had driven me to go to medical school. The people who had inspired me to go; I wrote about them in it too. Me and my interaction with them and how they impacted my life. My client was my biggest influence He is a pediatric orthopedic surgeon. He was older. He still works 6 days a week, 12 hour days and is going to be 70 years old next week, next year. He's an incredible person and he just loves his job so much and he's so good at it. The kids love him to death. It's just so sweet. That was a big part of it.

Q:
When did you get all your applications in? Did you apply to AMCAS early or late and then did you get the rest of yours in early or late?

A:
Wasn't the AMCAS deadline June 15th? I think I put mine in the middle of July.

Q:
So, pretty early? Do you think that helped you?

A:
They all said it would. I don't think it hurt me. They told me not to take the August MCAT, that it would handicap the time. So I didn't do that. I wish I had though because then I would have had organic. If my scores had been really awful, I would have taken them over in August. But I was concerned about that handicapping your file kind of thing. So if you take it over in August, then you don't get the luxury of an early application.

Q:
How many schools did you apply to?

A:
Eleven. Six in Chicago, five out of Chicago.

Q:
How did you choose the others?

A:
Locale, name and type of school. In that order — location, name, and then type of school.

B:
Tell me about your secondary applications.

Q:
They were awful. I'd like to just preface all of it by saying that applying to medical school is worse than all of medical school so far. It was a terrible experience. I sent secondaries back. I tried to get them in on time or within the 2 weeks or so like they say to do. But it was almost impossible to lead your normal life, fill out all those applications, have people read them and then change them

and have some more people read them. It just got to be such a
headache that although I slaved over the first 2 or 3, by the middle
of the pile, I was just like, yeah, that sounds good to me.

I did have a good friend of mine, who was a superb writer
and a big critic, read my work through the whole thing. And he
said, by the end, I had become a very good writer.   So it did
improve my writing ability. It gets better by the end. So my sug-
gestion there would be save the ones that you really want to go to
as late as you can. Although they send back those things as soon
— you want to get the secondaries back quick, but I wouldn't do
those first. If you want to go to a specific school, I wouldn't do that
school's first because it's going to sound bad. Unless you use the
same essays for everybody. I don't know if everyone improves like
I improved, but it was significantly different.

Q:
How did you choose the people that you got to send recommendations for you and who did you choose?

A:
It wasn't very hard because you have a maximum of six recommendations that you can get for the most part. You have to have
one from a chemistry professor. I don't know if everybody else
knows, but this is what I was told. I don't even know who told me
that, but it could have been my chemistry professor who was the
hardest one to get it in the first place. Also, I had one from my
anatomy professor at U of M who was my counselor at U of M who
told me not to go to medical school. So I had one from him, had
one from my old boss. I had one from my client who inspired me
to go, who was a physician.   So that covered both my academic
life and my professional life.

Q:
For your interviews, what were the different types of interviews you
had, as far as styles?

A:
I only interviewed at 3 schools in Chicago and one didn't interview
at all. The Rush interview — we had an interview with an attending and you had an interview with an admissions person.   Both
went great. The admissions guy tried to sell me on their new curriculum.   He did such a good job that I decided to go to
Northwestern. I didn't want the new curriculum. I didn't think it
was a good idea. I didn't want a new way of learning, I kind of

liked the old way! And he was so excited about it that it just sound-
ed like a good idea, except they don't have any lecture. And I was
still a little nervous about the whole no lecture theory. I had a
friend in the program there — she said it was great.

Q:
Do you remember any specifics about your interviews?

A:
I remember I glanced down at my file at Rush and I recognized the
guy's name who had reviewed my file. He had worked with me on
a chart; he was my consultant so I knew him. And I don't know if
it was a coincidence there that he reviewed my chart or my file. I
knew he had reviewed my file, but it was just weird that out of all
the people that sit on the admissions board he was there. He had
no idea that I was coming to medical school.
        For the interview at Northwestern, they had the panel
interview. I thought that was very cool. I had a great experience
with it.

Q:
Now if you could just reiterate general recommendations for somebody applying for medical schools.

A:
Take your MCAT early. I know it sounds bad, you don't want to
waste any more time than possible, but take it in August the year
before you apply. Take all your classes first. It sounds stupid, but
it's true. Don't be put off by the other students — what they've
done, where they're going, how many times they've taken the class
over, whatever. Don't even listen to them. And the same kind of
goes for the counselors. I don't think they know what's going on.

Q:
How about the whole decision to go back to school?

A:
Consider it very heavily. I think the best thing to do is to immerse
yourself in the world of medicine as much as possible beforehand.
Because once you go — I don't know how most people pay for it,
but personally, I'm on loans. I can't quit. After one year of school,
I'm pretty much in it for life. That alone frightens me, makes me
warn others that it's a serious decision. It's like stepping off with

both feet, one big 'ol jump. It's like, oh, I really want to do this.
Cool, you're going. Nobody drops out the second year.

Q:
Thanks a lot Margy.

Interview Six — Lisa Stranc

LISA STRANC: Lisa is twenty-eight years old. She majored in Psychology and graduated from Loyola University while working full time.

Q:
What you did before coming to medical school? Tell me something about your undergrad and work experience.

A:
During college I worked many jobs. I worked in an office supply store, in a garden center, a drug rehab hospital, for an insurance company, and finally, as a psychiatric technician. The job at the insurance company was my longest standing job and I did that for about four years. My boss there worked with me when I decided to start going to school full time. He was very flexible and let me cut back my hours at work. They were extremely supportive of me there. The job at the drug and alcohol rehab hospital was a good thing to have on my application, and so was my last job that I had before entering medical school—the psych tech position at a psychiatric hospital.

I started school at Oakton Community College, about a year and a half after high school. I worked full time and took one or two courses at a time for about three years, and finally got through one year of undergraduate study. I knew I wanted to study psychology so that's what I majored in. At that time, I had no plans for medical school at all.

I worked full time for about seven years while continuing school part time. It wasn't until my eighth year that I went to school full time. The last three or four years were at Loyola University. That's where I graduated from and it was there, at Loyola, that I decided to go to medical school. I had always been a psych major, but I never wanted to be a psychologist. But I really like working with people and I figured no matter what field I chose, psychology would be a useful tool.

You can get either a B.S. or a B.A. in psychology, and I was fortunate enough to have an advisor who steered me into the science part of psychology This made my transition to pre med a little bit easier. It wasn't until I started taking some science courses and ended up with some excellent teachers at Loyola, especially in biology, that I became interested in medical school. So, I took the premedical courses as electives, and got my degree in psychology.

Q:
Did you have any method in choosing your courses and teachers?

A:
No. I really didn't have much of a choice because I took only the basics—a year of bio, a year of general chem, o chem, physics, and calculus—and I just signed up for what fit best into my schedule. But when it came time for second semester I had a better idea of which teachers to take, and I also had a less stringent schedule because I cut my hours at work.   But the only teacher that I was able to retain for a second semester was my physics teacher. I wanted to stick with the same professor that I had for first semester because I thought he was great. A lot of the students didn't like him and were out of there after the first semester which I thought was kinda funny, but he was tough and he really challenged me. I wanted to stay with that teacher because, finally, after so much struggling, physics came together for me and I finally understood what I was doing. I really did struggle a lot through the first semester though. But I worked closely with that teacher. He knew me and he knew how I thought, and he was incredibly personally challenging.

Q:
O.K. And how many courses did you take at a time, in general? Science courses?

A:
Science courses? One. But I went through summer school, too. So I would take, for example, organic chem during the summer with a lab. It was only the last year and a half of college that I went full time, so other than that time, I worked full time and took two or three classes.

Q:
Sure, so you had a full load besides that. Say, four other classes, or two other classes. How did you study for your courses?

A:
For some of the science courses, I think it was only bio, I used to tape the lectures because I thought that was a really good way for me to study. That way I could concentrate on what the professor was saying in class and I didn't have to worry about not taking notes frantically. Then I would take the tapes and go outside in the sun to sunbathe, plug in the tape, and study. And it was a really

passive way of learning but, for me it worked really well. Other than that, I thought it was very important to get old tests. In organic chemistry they were made available for us.

I did not study in study groups. I was not somebody that could study well with other people because I like to talk. And other people got mad. So I learned really quick that I couldn't study in study groups.

Q:
Tell me about your advisor that you used.

A:
I had an advisor when I first started at Loyola that was pretty instrumental in guiding me into medicine. I think she somehow understood that I didn't really have a direction and she took that lead and led me into the science part of psychology. I think she also believed that I could do more than I thought I could. So, she was pretty instrumental in telling me to take classes that were more challenging. For example, I wanted to stop at algebra and she told me to take calculus. So she pushed me to challenge myself educationally. And then for the medical school applications, I used our premed advisor but solely for political reasons. I didn't really want to do that, but I did because medical schools asked you who your advisor is, and If you didn't use that advisor they want to know why.

Q:
Tell me about your extra-curricular activities.

A:
As I said, for the most part I worked full time and went to school part time, but in addition to that, I did some volunteer work. And, I think the volunteer work really helped with my application to med school because I had a long history of it. I graduated high school in '86 and started volunteering at various things in '87 all the way through to when I applied to med school. And I think that medical schools interpreted that long-term volunteer work at as being indicative of me being serious about what I wanted to do and serious about wanting to help people. Some of the things that I did were totally non-medically related. The Run-Away Switchboard was one of the first things I did here in Chicago. I was also on an Addictions Awareness team, I taught Sunday School for 4-year olds, and participated in the Special Olympics as an instructor/volunteer.

Also I trained my dog at North Shore Dog Training School.

I think that even things like that are very important for med school applications. Medical school committees want to know that you are dedicated to something or have a responsibility to someone or something, and so I definitely included that on my app. Some other things that I did that were more medically related was volunteer for Open Hand Chicago, a Meals-On-Wheels service for people with AIDS which delivers hot and cold meals to people who are home bound with AIDS and can't get out to the store. That was actually one of the most challenging things that I've done as a volunteer. Also for two years I was a patient representative at St. Francis Hospital. Once a week, sometimes twice a week for maybe two to three hours and I was assigned to a floor and I'd go around and talk to patients. I got a lot of insight from patients about what it's like to be in the hospital, and when I was doing some of the interviews at med schools I used a lot of the examples from my experiences as a patient representative. They'd say, "How do you know you're going to be able to relate to a patient." And, I could cite a specific example, "Well, there was this one patient I visited...." Or I could say "I know how to listen to patients. Here's an example." It helps to have concrete examples.

Q:
What about MCAT? When do you think you should take it? How did you study for it?

A:
Take it in spring. For sure. I took Kaplan and I signed up for the one right before the MCAT. I applied for a financial scholarship for Kaplan because it's extraordinarily expensive, like $900. So I asked them if there was any kind of scholarship for people who couldn't afford it and there was. I had to give a letter of recommendation from the Dean and maybe some past taxes, and school financial aid letters and they gave me a full ride there at Kaplan which was helpful. The only thing I found really beneficial about Kaplan was taking the practice test and I did that on my own. I did not go to a lot of classes but it was beneficial to take the old test and then to review the questions I got wrong. So Kaplan helped a little bit.

Q:
And did you organize your studying around Kaplan?

A:
I hate to say it but I kinda crammed for the MCAT. I know that you're not supposed to do that but I did cram and I think I spent

most time on verbal reasoning. One because I was good at it, better at that than bio. Reasoning for me has been more of a strong point than memorizing. And two, for me, a test strategy was to learn how to pull the answers from the passages rather than spending all my time memorizing things, which I wasn't very good at doing. It worked.

Q:
How long did you study for the MCAT?

A:
I'd say I started studying about three weeks before.

Q:
Tell me about the non-essay and essay parts of your AMCAS application.

A:
For the AMCAS application, I stressed my work history that I had been self supporting ever since high school. Also, in the essay part I explained how work gave me experience that could be beneficial for medical school. For example, I explained that I worked and went to school and I did some volunteer work, and then I was able to say, "See, I can juggle different things. I can handle a stressful schedule." And also I stressed specific work incidences, like that I worked at a psych hospital, and I was able to call on experiences there to use as concrete examples for med school.

Q:
How did you apply for the fee waivers for AMCAS?

A:
I didn't have a lot of money. I certainly did not have money to apply to the number of schools that I applied to. So I applied for a waiver, and I think I needed to include my tax information and a financial aid statement from school. Once I got the waiver through AMCAS usually I could send copies of that waiver along with my secondary applications and most of my secondary application fees were also waived. Without that wavier, I would not have been able to apply to medical school.

Q:
On to your essay. What did you write about?

A:

For the essay, I talked about putting myself through school, again focusing on work and also I included my reasons for applying for medical school, why I wanted to be a doctor, and I just used my experience to back it up. I said, "This is why I want to go into medicine. I want to work with people and I have worked with people and this is how come I know that this is something I want to do." It's not just something that I've wanted to do all my life, it's something that evolved, and it is due to the experiences that I decided to go to med school.

Q:

Tell me about your secondary application.

A:

I wanted to make the general impression that I was different from the ordinary med school applicant and I wanted to stress that. One, because I felt like I was, but also because I thought it was beneficial to stand out. I thought that my experience, not only what I experienced in the work field, but also having to juggle things—an apartment, the bills , the dog, and being independent and taking classes—I felt like being able to juggle those kind of real life things set me apart from other medical students. That's the impression that I wanted to portray in my secondary applications.

Q:

And did you update your application?

A:

I did update some of my applications with final grades and, when I did that, I usually included a little bit of extra information about what I was presently doing which was working at a psych hospital as a psychiatric technician. I included that because it was directly relevant and I thought that they would like that. I thought it would add to my application so I did include that. I think it is very important if there is any new information like that to keep sending it in. It shows that you're interested. There were some schools that I did not send the extra information to because I decided that I didn't want to go there and I ended up not getting into those schools. It could have been coincidence but I really think that if they see that you're sending extra information then obviously you are still interested.

Q:
Do you think timing is important when you're applying?

A:
I think timing is very important. I think the earlier you apply the better your chances. I applied late, not that late though, I think it was the first week of September. But applying late is harder, too, you know, because you're watching your other friends get interviews and you haven't even heard from that school yet. And a lot of schools have rolling admissions, so I think it's very important to apply as early as you can.

Q:
O.K. How did you choose the schools that you applied to?

A:
I applied to about twenty schools and I had no idea what my chances were of getting in. I was completely clueless. And, then, only as time went on, you know, when I got my first secondary, I was like, "Wow, I can get a secondary!" Then when I got my first interview, I was ecstatic, and then I got my first acceptance. I really couldn't believe it. I truly didn't know where I stood.

Like everybody who was applying, I applied to a lot of schools and they ranged from easy to difficult to get into. Not really easy but easier, relatively speaking.

The cost of school really didn't weigh on my decisions of whether or not to apply because it was going to be all financial aid for me in any case, it wasn't going to be any out-of-pocket expense. I felt like what's the difference in being $150,000 in debt or $200,000 in debt.

So really, the cost of the school wasn't that important in influencing which schools I applied to. But when I started getting some acceptances then the decision about where to go became a little bit more complicated and that was because, for me, the number one issue became financial aid. I had no outside income other than my psych tech job, which was low paying, so I didn't have anything saved. I'd already been in debt for eight years of undergraduate work so, for me, the financial aid was extremely important. Now most schools, consider you dependent, because you are dependent when you are in medical school. Northwestern was the only Illinois schools that gave an opportunity for me to claim myself as an independent. The University of Wisconsin was another one. In order to do that, I had to prove that I was independent for two years, provide my tax information and, if I met the criteria, I could get the loans based on my income alone which was essentially zilch which meant that I could get all recommended loans for the full ride. Also Northwestern has that loan capping program which means that after a specific amount of money that you borrow in recommended loans, the school pays for the rest of your education.

So, location and school, and financial aid were my three main determinants on which school I was going to attend. Northwestern had the best financial aid package. And it was in Chicago which was good because that's where I lived, and it was a good school. So that's how I ended up going here.

Q:
Great. Tell me how you chose the people you got your recommendations from.

A:
The people that I got recommendations from. I heard a lot of other people say, "I'll just get one from the o chem teacher because he's good" or whatever, and yet they never established a relationship with that person. I didn't want to do that. I wanted to get recommendations from people who knew me. I thought that would be better. So with the one science course that I struggled through which was physics, and I took that professor for both semesters, and got a letter of recommendation from him. He knew me well because he worked closely with me and I was in his office asking questions and asking for help. So I got a letter of recommendation from him.

Some schools wanted two science recommendations, but I really didn't have two science professors that I thought could give me substantial recs, so what I did was I got one from my medical ethics philosophy. I minored in philosophy. When I asked her she said to me that in order to write a letter of recommendation I had to take another course from her, give her my personal statement, and write up a biographical sketch for her She was pretty demanding. I remember weighing whether I really wanted to do this at this time just to get a recommendation or if I should just ask somebody else. I decided to go with her and so I gave her all that information and she ended up writing the best letter of recommendation for me. She spent a lot of time on that letter. So, that was a good decision. And then for the third rec, instead of using a second science like I was supposed to, I got one from my boss who was the president of the insurance company. I asked him to write a letter of recommendation for me, again, to solidify my work experience and how I did out in the work place.

I called some schools like Loyola who wanted two science recommendations and I said, "I haven't really taken that many science
courses and my professors didn't know me well. I have one, but
can I make my second science rec one from work instead?" And,
they said that was fine. So schools are pretty flexible and, as long
as you call and ask. I think it was better to have somebody who
knew me and work ethic very well, rather than a professor who did-
n't know me at all.

Q:
Let's go on to your interviews.

A:
My interviews?   Well to start with I wore a blue suit. I saw some
women wearing black and I thought it looked a little too bank-like
and then I saw some red and I didn't think that was good either. I
think, a blue suit is non threatening so that's what I wore for every
interview.

    I think the interview questions were fair. I guess I was pre-
pared for some sexist questions like how could you as a woman
want to be a doctor and what about kids and things like that. But
I didn't get anything like that at all. Since, I was prepared for those
so I think the questions in the interviews seemed relatively easy
compared to what I expected. Also, most every interview had
some ethical component and, if they didn't, or if it was small, I
often tried to create ethical questions because I had a background
in medical ethics and I liked to argue. I could take either side of an
ethical question. The answers that I think they liked were answers
that showed that you could see both sides. They weren't as interested in your answer, per se, they were more interested in how you
derived your answer and that you could see both sides of a situation. You could see and acknowledge and argue both sides of the
dilemma.

    And, also most of the questions that were asked I tried to
back up with experience. When they asked me "how would you
relate to a patient that was your age or, say, traumatically injured or
whatever". With my experience, I could probably pull something
from some instance that was somewhat related to what they were
talking about.   I'd say, "Well, you know I did once work with a
patient who was near my age who was traumatically injured and
blah, blah, blah." and I'd talk about how it was difficult or easy to
work with that person. I think it really helped to have concrete
examples.

Q:
And the different types of interviews?

A:
I did not like the panel interview. I only had one. I didn't like it because I felt like it was less personal. I felt like the interviewers were in more control of the interview and I wanted to have the opportunity to show that I was a little bit different. And, I felt like I was swallowed up in the panel interview. The single interview I liked better because I felt there was more freedom to be expressive. The student interviews I did not like, because they were too busy, you know, and they didn't seem to care as much.

Q:
Did you prepare for your interviews?

A:
No. I had interviewed for jobs and things like that so I have always felt pretty comfortable with interviews.

Q:
How about general recommendations?

A:
I would say the most important thing is experience, no matter what it is, just to let them know that you've done something other than school work and books. Experience, volunteer work, regular paid work, something that's related to the medical field, no matter what it is. I think, in answering any kind of question, it helps to back things up because they want to know that you've had some kind of experience with it, and, that you're not just giving an answer because it is the correct answer to give or because you think it's what they want to hear. But, rather, this is what your experience has been and this is how you think that can be beneficial in apply-ing to medical school and in getting through medical school.

     I remember an interviewer asked me, "Are you really will-ing to put in the long hours it takes to be a doctor. Why don't you be a nurse?" And, I said, "You know, I AM willing to put in the long hours. I know that I'm willing because I once worked full time and took three classes and did everything else that I needed to do in my life. And that was a lot longer day than I put in now just working full time. So yes, I know that I can do it, that I am willing and capa-ble of putting in the time and whatever it takes to be a doctor. And he was completely satisfied with that. So, I think experience is the best thing for someone who is applying to medical school.

Q:
Excellent. Thanks, Lisa.

Interview Seven — Steve Herwick

STEVE HERWICK: Steve is twenty-seven years old. He graduated from Northwestern University with a degree in Political Science. He then worked as a marketing and fund-raising manager for the Museum of Broadcast Journalism in Chicago.

Q:
Tell me a little bit about what you did as an undergrad, what you majored in, and then what you did afterwards.

A:
As an undergrad, I didn't really know what I wanted to do when I went to college at first, and I ended up majoring in political science because I had a strong interest in it. But after a while, after a few years, I realized that I kind of missed the more natural science type stuff. So I wasn't sure that I wanted to go back to school. And it took a few years away from it to realize that I probably would want to go back. So I graduated with a political science degree with very little in the way of natural sciences or anything that I would have needed in that respect.

So once I graduated, I got a job at a museum basically doing fund raising stuff, development for the museum. I did that for about a year while I was looking into different post-bacc. premed programs, just kind of researching how I would need to go about applying to medical school and gaining admission. And making sure that's what I wanted to do before putting the time and the money and the effort into it.

So I worked there for about a year. I finally chose a program to go back to and set my course schedule and made a whole time schedule. Then I changed jobs to something I could work around my classes, and it happened to be for a small medical practice. And it was basically office type work...the business end of medicine. It was really helpful in that I got to meet a lot of doctors that could show me things that you don't necessarily get to experience from the outside.   So I did that while I was taking my classes.

Q:
What courses did you take?

A:
I had to take everything first of all. So I took the chemistry and gen-

eral biology the first summer and then ended up taking organic and cell biology. I took more than I needed to so it was kind of a nice background. In fact I got an anatomy class in, in addition to physics and so forth that I needed to take. I did take biochemistry. I can't remember precisely what my schedule was but I remember I had anatomy and biochemistry, second semester organic all at one time. I guess I was technically full-time for one full school year just because it was actually cheaper to pay full-time than to pay for individual courses. That's why I was able to take some classes that I didn't necessarily need because the price was the same to be a full-time student where I was.

Q:
Did you have a specific method of choosing your professors?

A:
It was at a pretty small school. It was a very small liberal arts school that was really strong in basic science, and I think that was the best thing for me because if I had been at some big state school, I wouldn't have known what in the world to take or who to take. But everybody there was really interested in teaching, and all my instructors knew ,even if I was in classes with some of the under-grads , they all knew my situation. They knew you were doing it because you really were trying to learn the material. So that was kind of nice.

Q:
Tell me about your program.

A:
It was at this school, Illinois Benedictine College. It's in suburban Chicago. I was technically a post-baccalaureate student, so they do have a post-bacc program but it's not like some universities that have a post-bacc premed program that they set you in a track and they decide it all for you. Being a post-bacc student, I could get an advisor. Basically what I did is I went in and got an advisor. We worked together to work out a schedule and a timetable and that type of stuff. I was also able to speak to instructors before register-ing and say, "Listen, is this something that you think would help me given my situation?" So it was pretty loose in terms of what I need-ed to take outside of just preparing myself for the MCAT and other scheduling conflicts with work. I was in a degree program for what's called a second major. So you don't get a degree from the school, but you have what's considered a second major from the

college.

Q:
When you were taking your classes what materials were the most helpful to you to study? Did you study out of textbooks, old notes, old tests, study groups?

A:
Other than just the normal classroom materials that were given in the textbooks that were used by the instructors, I think the only thing that I'd never really done before that I found really helpful was to study in small groups. I don't think that would have been possible or as easy if it were a big program where I didn't know the people. Basically I knew everybody in all the classes, because it was a small enough school that everybody that was taking an upper level biochemistry and organic chemistry was for the most part in the same classes. So you could get into little study groups, and that was helpful. I hadn't really done that as an undergrad, so it was kind of nice.

Q:
You said you were assigned an advisor. You sound like you used the advisor. Did you use him to both help you schedule your classes and plan your applications?

A:
 When I was working at the museum I was trying to figure out how I was going back to school basically having no science background. I talked to advisors at several different schools in the area when I trying to figure out how I wanted to do it, where I wanted to go, and what was the best way to do it.

Q:
Advisors from medical school or from premedical programs?

A:
Premed programs and some medical programs. It's hard to contact people at medical schools sometimes. They've got X number of undergrads from across the country trying to get in good with people who make decisions, and it's hard get phone calls returned. People who are premed advisors are generally pretty good, and they know what you need to do. They know when you need to have stuff done by, they're used to counseling people to get into schools so they know what are things you want to avoid, that type

of thing. So I must have talked to people at 5 or 6 different schools, some of which had set post-bacc programs, some of which didn't. I actually found out that a lot of people were more than willing to talk about that kind of stuff. Every school that I approached, I could find somebody that was really helpful.

Q:
Did your program have a central processing committee that wrote you a letter?

A:
Yeah, they did. At this school, most of the instructors knew you anyway because there's a core of faculty that teach the upper level sciences . You interviewed with five different faculty members and they all conducted the interview however they wanted to do it. And then they meet and write a letter based on your performance at the school and consider your background. It was very much like a medical school application because you had to write an essay for them, interview with five of the faculty members, and then they met and decided how they wanted to recommend you. That was really nice because then I really didn't have to worry about getting a bunch of recommendations from people. I still had one from my advisor in undergrad, but a lot of med school applications said either send three recommendations or a committee recommenda-tion. So what I usually did was send the committee one and then my one from undergrad.

Q:
Tell me a little bit about your extracurricular activities and what you did first of all that was medically related and then non-med-ically related.

A:
I didn't do all together too much because of the fact that I was working full-time while I was taking my classes. My work in the medical practice consisted of billing. And it was flexible enough that I didn't need to be there during their office hours. I could go in whenever I wanted to and do it. So I'd usually spend a full day there Saturday, go in a little bit on Sunday and then mornings until early afternoon, and then go to a few classes in the afternoon. It was definitely busy for a little while. But in the long run, it made a year's worth of difference, maybe even two, just because I could get the classes under my belt that I needed.

Q:
Have you done some medically-related activities?

A:
I can't think of anything. No, not really. I definitely had exposure, but nothing that I've gone out of my way to do. Yeah, just because my father's a doctor. I'd sometimes just go in with him, not necessarily see patients, but just had a little bit of background in terms of lifestyle. To tell you the truth, that's the thing that kept me from going into medicine in the first place. I just wanted to avoid it. When you get out of high school and you're a decent student and people know your father's a doctor, they just assume, "of course he's going to go to med school." So it was maybe a little bit of rebellion against that expectation.

Q:
Let's talk about the AMCAS application.

A:
I just remember having a hell of time fitting all that stuff on the spaces, I mean typing in the squares. I don't really remember having too much trouble condensing the stuff. The one thing I remember doing was photocopying the stuff and just typing rough copies just to get the spacing down because that was so hard to do. Because if you had just typed everything out...I mean figuring out what you can abbreviate was a big ...that took up a lot of time. Sometimes you have to change the spacing on the typewriter just to get certain things in the spaces. In fact I remember my essay, I had to get it professionally printed because it took from the very top to the very bottom of that space they give you, and I couldn't find a typewriter that held it steady to type the last couple of lines, so I had to take it to a printer.

Q:
As far as your essay, what did you write about?

A:
Basically, I just explained my rationale for putting this effort and money and time into going back to school and why it was something that I kind of drifted away from for a little while and what drove me back to it.

Q:
I'm sure you filled out a number of secondary applications. What

was your general impression of those and how did you use them to your advantage?

Q:

A:
I honestly can't think of anything extraordinary that I put on them. Having worked at the museum for a little while, I had worked on a couple of big projects where I had people working under me that were always good to talk about. Even if somebody was looking for some type of accomplishment or something, I put standard stuff on essays. I didn't write about trips to the Himalayas or anything. I stuck to my background.

Q:
Did you update your applications after that? Did you send schools extra material?

A:
Yeah, I sent grade reports just because I was continuing to take classes. I had one semester of classes come in and another summer class that I was taking come in.

Q:
Did you apply early or late?

A:
I got all my AMCAS stuff in pretty early. You know the deadline is in June, and I got it in the end of June, but I knew that I couldn't take the MCAT until the Fall because I was taking physics over that last summer, so it was kind of incomplete. Most of the schools wouldn't even send me secondaries until they got the MCAT because they just considered your file open. That was kind of frustrating. It was a little nerve-wracking. I was thinking about even taking the MCAT without having had physics. Just doing a little brush-up on my own which probably would have been stupid. I kept hearing from so many people that, "oh, you have to take the early MCAT. You're killing yourself if you don't," but I guess it was all right. It turned out OK. But I definitely think you really need to have the other part in early at least. I don't think they want to hear about somebody for the first time in November. I think they want to maybe get an application, see that it's good enough not to total-ly disregard, and then just wait for your scores to come in.

Q:
How many schools did you apply to?

A:
I applied to 13 schools.   I applied to all the schools in my state which is seven. Beyond that, there were a few other schools that I was really interested in for one reason or another. Some schools that I thought would be easy to get into or having talked to advisors they said were pretty easy to get into. I guess I had no idea how I was going to look to an admissions committee. I didn't know if somebody was going to say, "oh my god, we have to get him," or if I was just going to be on every wait list or if I wasn't going to have a chance. I really didn't know, so I figured I needed to get a lot of them out.

Q:
You obviously got some interviews. What were some general impressions on your interviews?

A:
The one thing that I found when I went on interviews was that I felt a lot older than the other applicants even though I was only 3 years older. Usually before you have an interview, you're sitting in this room with the other applicants and there are all these kids in suits that don't fit them. Everybody just seems like they're all dressed up and they don't look right and they look nervous and out of place. I think the most important thing is to just be entirely natural. I just felt that these people just had so much more stress than they needed to have. I think that probably ended up being to my advantage. None of them were that bad, even the interviews that were the hardest, that had challenging questions, they really weren't all that bad. I think that the committee interviews that I had before my recommendations committee were intentionally harder than any med school interviews that I'd see.

Q:
Do you remember any specifics from your interviews?

A:
I think there are certain questions that I would go in prepared for. There are particular questions that you have to have answers right. Whether it's people that ask you, "well, why are you going into medicine knowing that the environment is changing so fast and the future's so uncertain, job security's uncertain?" and this and that. Why would you make this choice? There are certain questions that you have to have addressed before going in. Questions like "what would you do concerning health care reform?" Maybe only a cou-

ple of times it came up, but it's one of those things that you have to think about how you're going to answer.

Q:
What about ethical questions?

A:
You get a couple of ethical questions but I don't think any of them were all that bad. I do remember in one of my interviews for the recommendations committee, one of the interviewers would drill you with all these ethical questions and he'd try to back you into a corner and try to get you to contradict yourself. Don't let anyone do that to you even if they seem to be trying to do that. Just be confident in your responses. Nobody's going to think any less of you if you have an ethical viewpoint or moral viewpoint that's opposed to theirs, as long as you stick to it and seem to have a rationale for coming from where you are.

Q:
And then how did you choose the school that you wanted to go to or that you ended up going to?

A:
That was probably the hardest part. It came down to a lot of different factors that all kind of factor in, but I think in the long run, the reason I came here was that I liked the idea of the revised curriculum. I didn't like the idea of sitting in class for 8 hours a day. It had been a while since I'd just been taking classes all day long. I think that was the big thing for me.

Q:
Are there any other general recommendations that you would give to somebody who is a nontraditional student?

A:
I would definitely recommend talking to as many different people before trying to plan out your approach. As many different people in different areas, whether they're in medical school, advisors, undergraduate advisors, and so forth. Nobody's going to give you exactly the same answer but when you talk to enough of them you will know what you need to do. The first couple I talked to, I thought they knew exactly what they were talking about, but when you talk to a few more people that basically have the same position at a different school or from a slightly different background,

they'll tell you something else. You really have to figure out a little bit on your own exactly what you need to do.

Q:
That's good advice. Thanks Steve.

Interview Eight - Arturo Gutierrez

ARTURO GUTIERREZ: Arturo is twenty-nine and married. After graduating from Cornell University with an Engineering degree he worked as an engineer for two years. Later, he worked as a product management executive in consumer products, pharmaceuticals, and candy.

Q:
Tell me little bit about what you did before you came to medical school.

A:
I did a number of different things. I actually graduated from college in 1988 and although I was an engineer by degree, I ended up working in marketing. Actually I started in engineering back in '88 for a consumer products company and did manufacturing engineering for two years before transferring into their marketing department. And that was P& G, and so marketing was definitely the way to go in that company. And from there, I took off working for the next five years for a whirlwind of mostly Fortune 500 companies in product marketing.

I worked initially for P & G and when I got into their marketing department, they sent me to Cincinnati. You got to understand, I was also 22 or so, so I was very anxious to live. And I'd grown up in a sort of suburban hell of South Florida so I wanted to get out and see the world. So I got sick of Cincinnati predictably. And so I quit and worked for Bristol Myers Squibb in New York City in marketing. And all along, I kind of was interested in medicine, I just wasn't ready to make a commitment, and working for a drug company was sort of halfway for me to think about it. From there I went to work for Nestle which is in Glendale, in California outside of L.A., and did that for a while but got sick of that. I decided, Okay, I'm 26. I did a post-bacc program at Bryn Mawr College in Philadelphia. From there, I applied to school.

Q:
 So how did you actually make your decision? Was there a point where you decided you wanted to go to med school?

A:
Well, all along — I was always interested in it, but every time I'd consider it, I'd pick up an MCAT review book and put it back down

and say, forget this. I didn't have the organic chemistry ever, although I had plenty of physics. As an engineering major, I did very poorly, I was a slob as an undergrad. So that might be relieving to those who didn't have a stellar undergraduate performance. But I did have to do well in some biology courses and some chemistry courses to bolster my record.

It finally got to a point in my career in marketing — I'd look at the people who were one or two levels above me and I realized that I didn't want to do that. And I stopped thinking about the next two years where my interests were really just about making more money and having somewhat more responsibility, but just living fat in business. And I just realized that I didn't want to do that long-term. I had to bite the bullet, start all over, and do all this other stuff.

Q:
So, you enrolled in a post-bacc program?

A:
I applied to two. They're all over the place now but at the time, there were two big ones on the East Coast. And I was kind of an East Coast guy, even though I lived in LA for a little while. Columbia had a big program and Bryn Mawr had a really small program. Columbia came across, and I believe it was, very intense and competitive. Those dynamics kind of skewed me toward a smaller class. At Bryn Mawr it was 80 students versus 500.

I felt like I needed the full endorsement, recommendation, packaging of a formal post-bacc program. But in retrospect, had I not been that bad off, I would totally recommend and know a lot of people who did , taking the courses and doing well but not necessarily on such a formal, expensive level.

Q:
So can you expand a little more on the program?

A:
I learned a fair amount. At Bryn Mawr they made it a big point not to talk about grades, so they kind of fostered a laid-back environment So it was not too hard. I took a lot of good courses. I took my required courses. It went well. It was kind of tough because it was such a transitional year because I had given up everything. And I was giving it up for nothing because it was required and preparatory, but it was flying with your eyes closed at night with no instruments, and no guarantees. Psychologically it was very diffi-

cult and expensive.

Q:
As far as choosing your courses, were they chosen for you?

A:
They required — they were good about counseling students about what — and any person who's taking that kind of risk ought to pick up a book and read the Medical Criteria of Admissions. You know the AMCAS puts out that book. So I knew what I needed to take and they counseled you. But I had taken some bio courses and I had taken some chem courses, so I kind of didn't bother with it. I took more advanced bio courses. Instead of intro biology, I took genetics. Instead of physics, I took neurobiology . Most people I knew in the program were English majors and had no science background. So they took the basic structured curriculum.

Q:
When you were studying for your premed courses, what type of materials did you find most helpful?

A:
Mostly my lecture notes supplemented with the text. It wasn't a lot of lecture, but the main points. And I would follow along and supplement when I didn't understand the text. I didn't have any review books or any outside anything. I had no MCAT books at all. Even when I took the test, I had no MCAT book.

Q:
Did you use study groups at all?

A:
On very rare occasions, I'd get together with one or two other people that I was close to, but not routinely and not any particular people. So sort of yes, but not by ritual.

Q:
Did you find it most beneficial to study on your own?

A:
Yes, mostly because I didn't study much, so it was like the heat of the moment.

Q:
In a formal program like that, there was probably tutoring available. Did you use anything like that?

A:
No.   It was available informally through faculty and through the
TAs and you could always pay people. There were always bio
majors and biochem majors and physics majors. The undergraduate stuff just really wasn't that hard, fortunately. Otherwise, I
couldn't have done it.

Q:
How long did it take you?

A:
One calendar year. And that's what it typically takes people. In the
summer, they'll take intro chem, chem I, chem II, general or inorganic chemistry. And then in the fall, they would start with biology, physics and organic, two terms of all of those. So in the fall and
in the spring, they'd have bio I, bio II, organic I, organic II, physics
I and II. One calendar year. People who started in the fall started
obviously not with organic chemistry, but with general chemistry.
And then in the next summer, they'd take organic, but that put them
at a disadvantage because they'd have to take the MCAT at some
point. And if they were going to take it in April, they couldn't really take it then because they didn't have any organic. And you
know that's a big component.

Q:
As far as advisement goes, did you use a school advisor to plan
your classes?

A:
Not so much the classes, but just to tell me if my thoughts were rea-
sonable. For instance, I wanted to take the MCAT in April. And
even though I was in organic chemistry, my biology was eleven
years old. So I talked to my advisor about that as well as the
advantages of April versus August MCAT. I showed my AMCAS
essay to her and got her feedback. She was very helpful.

Q:
Tell me about your medical and non-medical extracurricular activities.

A:
Well, when I worked in marketing, there were over-the-counter drugs that I worked on. So I had to understand somewhat how they worked, although that wasn't as critical — a little bit about medical, clinical sciences for instance. At one point, I worked on some itch product for your skin and understanding how a clinical comparison or a clinical trial is done between two products. I learned because I didn't know much about it, plus I had to learn a lot of the regulatory aspects of federal monographs and all the things that the FDA lays down in regard to drugs. And although they exist for prescription drugs, obviously, they're maybe even more stringent with over-the-counter drugs because they are the only stopgap. Whereas, theoretically MDs stand between the consumer and the prescription drugs.

I learned all that stuff in marketing, plus when I was in the post-bacc year I worked part-time, like 20-25 hours a week, as a mental health counselor. Which meant I'd sit in a halfway house, dole out medication, and talk to schizophrenics for most nights. I would encourage people that they could handle it, and it kept the light at the end of the tunnel there for me. Although I may not be a psychiatrist at some point, it's still contact with patients in sort of a clinical setting. There's all this crap going through your mind as a premedical student-none of it seems relevant — what the hell does organic chemistry have to do with being a doctor? The answer is, not much. In fact, not at all. But, it sort of gave me some reason to pursue it, and it also looked good on applications that I worked as and I was paid as a counselor.

Q:
Did you do any volunteer activities?

A:
I had done some volunteer work when I was in business. Things like Big Brothers. I was the philanthropy chair in my fraternity. I was a mentor for some youth collaboration organization. This was all in different cities.

Q:
That's good. Now we're going to talk a little bit about the MCAT. Do you have any recommendations about when to take it?

A:
April. If at all possible, the early one I think is helpful. And I'm basing that not only on my personal experience, but pairing my

experience and my scores and my invitations to interview, with other people that all else being equal, may be even better off in terms of the MCAT, who took it in August. It just makes all the difference. And I think that's well-documented in the "So, you Want to Get Into Med School" books which aren't written for non-traditional students.

Q:
How did you prepare for the MCAT?

A:
I really didn't study. A week before the MCAT, I started to freak out. And I stopped going to my classes. It was bad. Literally I'm not exaggerating. For a week, I broke out my old physics book and started skimming chapters. I had a bio book and the organic chemistry was fresh in my mind, as was the general chemistry, because I took all of those within the previous ten months. So I just had to brush up on those things that were ten or twelve years old. So I would highly recommend that people not do that. It was just not worth it mentally too because I was just a mess those last few weeks.

Q:
How would you recommend organizing your studying for the MCAT?

A:
If you have a pretty comfortable understanding of what you're learning, don't let what other people do freak you out, and that applies to undergrad, MCAT , med school, life. It's a struggle because it's very easy to get caught up and do the whole yardstick thing, how tall am I compared to that person rather than just how I'm learning this stuff. But that's human nature. So it's highly variable. I know other people who studied maybe a little more than I did — these people that got 13s and 14s on their MCAT.

Q:
Your AMCAS application, on your non-essay part, how did you prioritize what you thought you should list?

A:
I stayed more current. I embellished at the expense of the other things, more that was more related. I talked more about my drug marketing experience. Like the fact that at one point, I was on a

multi-functional team — looking at which drug the company should pursue given the success of a lot of previous brands like Ibuprofen and other things that were once over-the-counter. I'd talk about that more than I'd talk about that I'd developed a 45-million dollar advertising campaign for Pampers. Which is a much bigger business accomplishment than sitting on a crusty, old team of MDs and PhDs. I made it sound a little bit more medical. I focused more on those issues and volunteer activities that were more related to medicine, although there weren't that many. And I think that's just common sense for people.

Q:
In your essay, what did you talk about?

A:
I talked about ... it was so cheesy, but my faculty advisor thought it was the right way to go. Just about my life-long desire to be a physician and why I wanted to be one, which is a very standard-type thing. You feel so cheesy writing about these things sometimes. But if you have a compelling story to tell and you can tell it in a way that doesn't sound too self-aggrandizing or too self-important or too mushy, then you ought to tell it because they're interested in hearing about it. In particular, if you had some barriers, which all non-traditional students have to get there, include them because it shows them that you are really interested in this field, that it's not just a haphazard decision, and you're willing to make sacrifices to attain it. And from their point of view, they want to know you are enduring because they don't want to bring in people that can't make it.

For those reasons, I sort of agreed with my advisor even though I hated writing about me, me, me. All my motivations. Family influences. I had to reconcile the fact that, what the hell was I doing? There were seven years in between graduation and me being a candidate for their school. It was just a matter of explaining to them and being honest about not being ready to make the commitment. While I found this career in business rewarding financially, I didn't find it personally rewarding. And I think that that reconciliation helped. I got lots of interviews and things went pretty well for everything that went against me, like my grades and my solid, but not by any means spectacular, MCATs.

I don't think that I was given interviews that I didn't deserve, but I think that the essay and being a non-traditional student can come to your advantage if you package it correctly. And you explain things confidently, but not self-consciously. It's easy to get self-conscious about your undergraduate grades or the fact that your whole purpose for 5 or 6 years was to make money or the people that say worked in law or something that has nothing to do with it, to explain that you really are genuine and you want to do this for the right reasons. It can be an advantage.

Q:
Tell me about your secondary applications.

A:
Because there was so much about my record and background that you just can't fit onto an AMCAS, the secondary applications gave me the space to expand on my background. Northwestern, it's the perfect example. They wanted you to write about examples when you showed leadership, examples where you communicated an initiative to some people and led them to get there. I think schools really do want people with some leadership skills, some communication skills, and a little bit of maturity. If they give you an opportunity to write an essay about that, and you've got some salient experience, go gangbusters on it and just push it. You don't have to sound like you were hot shit in your previous life, but that you are capable of handling responsibility and organizing people and thoughts, being a leader.

All those things they want after they know you can cut it in their academics. All those secondaries are a great opportunity to do that. Not all of them ask for that type of information. Some of them might say attach a resume, and that's a great opportunity or maybe you send one anyway. I don't think for your secondaries you ever get penalized for providing too much information. If you have a CV or a resume send it. Some people send additional letters of recommendation. I didn't do that. But once you get to secondaries, it's a good sign.

Q:
And when did you apply?

A:
The first day that AMCAS was accepting applications. That's the biggest advantage of taking the April MCAT. You can apply early. It's just timing. June 15 .   But I had given up so much and I was so frazzled by the prospect of not knowing what to do next if I didn't get in that I didn't take a chance. I was anal retentive. Which was very against my mode of studying. As much as I might be a slacker, I wasn't about to be laid-back about those kind of things. I

wasn't going to miss a single deadline. I wasn't going to do anything at the last minute. I was going to be the first one of the first dozen at the door.

I've seen it written that the main advantage of taking this exam in April — you go through a lot of turmoil to do it because you're taking classes, chances are. And you're not as ready because you didn't have the whole summer to prepare yourself. If you're going to go through all that grief and you finally get back your scores, you're OK with them, you damn well better take advantage of it. Otherwise, what's the point? I don't know anybody who took it in April and then waited until August or later to send it in.

Q:
OK, tell me about how you chose the schools that you applied to.

A:
About a dozen.

Q:
How did you select those schools?

A:
I probably started with parts of the country I would want to live in. So I didn't even consider schools in states or cities that had absolutely no appeal. Part of that was knowing that by then I was getting married and my spouse was going to have to be reasonably happy there because she's not a student. And we're both city people anyway. Most if not all of them were in large cities. You could apply to a dozen schools just between say Philadelphia and Chicago or Philadelphia and New York. Beyond that I kind of looked for a range of difficulty getting in, reputation, published typical MCAT scores, and other factors like number of in state applicants accepted versus out of state applicants accepted. So I kind of spread it across from couple of reach schools, to a couple that I thought might be gimmes.

Q:
Did you apply to both public and private?

A:
Yes. I was a New York state resident then. The SUNY system has a number of schools and they're significantly cheaper.

Q:
Did you choose by the cost of the school?

A:
In as much that state versus the private. But all the private schools, once you're talking about those, you're talking about a fortune and you're splitting hairs between $24,000 and $22,000.

Q:
Did you apply to any non-AMCAS schools?

A:
Yes I did.   A number of them don't participate in the standard AMCAS application. You apply directly to them.   I applied to Rochester, Harvard, Columbia. In fact, Rochester and Harvard didn't even require the MCAT. Columbia is a great school and it's in New York. We were living in New York City. There were a number of other things that went into the decisions.   But then in thinking about it, whether you get in or not, you consider a lot of other things like the location within the location.   For example, Albert Einstein is in New York City. It's in the middle of nowhere Bronx versus Cornell, upper East side, or NYU versus Columbia.   But Columbia's not that bad, it's just scary.   So things like neighborhood within the neighborhood, how competitive is it and that's really hard to assess the feel, and even some of the ones I applied to were pressure cookers.   For example, Cornell. I'm really glad I didn't get in there because I might have gone and I'd have really ended up hating it.

Q:
Okay. How did you choose the people who wrote recommendations for you?

A:
Just my relationships with them. And also their status. I mean I wasn't going to get a TA to write one, a post-doctoral, somebody that wasn't on the faculty.   Bryn Mawr was so small that there weren't that many choices and one of them was the faculty director. One of them was something like that in chemistry. But more importantly than that were people that I actually had an opportunity to interact with and ask questions to, because I asked a lot of questions. That's how I learn — I don't like to just sit there and read the book. I ask a lot of questions, even if I look stupid because that way I'll learn it and I won't be stupid. So that and most important-

ly because otherwise you're just going to get a form letter. That doesn't do you any good either. A form letter from even some of the upper level management where I used to work might be impressive for business purposes, but not very helpful because they don't know you well.

Q:
What was your impression of having all your information in one place?

A:
The way I remembered this was the profs and the non-profs would send these things to Bryn Mawr. Then the Bryn Mawr dean would compile and create a little dossier of all these letters and her summary of what everybody says. And what they do is, you tell them what schools you're applying to because you can never see your recommendations and they take your packet and send it to the schools. From what I heard from people they did an impressive, very good job of — and I don't know if that meant the organization of it, that it looked really good and it was well presented or the content. Hopefully it was both. But it struck me as minimally the organization; it was well-organized, the letters were there and in order that they thought were more important and they were summarized and packaged well.

Q:
And they wrote a summary letter.

A:
Yeah. The Dean. Basically the premed advisor who was the Associate Dean of some sort wrote a cover letter that summarized her impressions working with the student and what the faculty said. Even though they are going to read what the faculty said, that summary was just sort of as an abstract — here's what you're looking at with this student. And I had a good relationship with her. I think that's helpful to get to know people, in addition to the profs who are going to write them, if there's anybody who's going to write a department letter or a college letter get to know the person well. And you can do that in a genuine way — you're asking questions, you're getting to know them, you're giving opinions. You're not just sitting there trying to brown-nose with the person.

Q:
It sounds like during your classes you went to your professors and

you asked questions. Is that right?

A:

Yes. It was a small, very atypical very artsy-type of environment that allowed that. In fact, Bryn Mawr is an all-women's college undergrad. My point is that it was small and so de-emphasizing of grades and accomplishments and more focused on learning, it actually was an environment conducive to doing that. And it was helpful because I learned a lot and because they got to know me. They were able to write better letters.

Q:

Would you recommend that program?

A:

I would. It's expensive, If you don't think you're going to get in without a structured program, then it's money well-spent.

Q:

Tell me about your interview experiences.

A:

They were good. I had some experience interviewing working for all those companies and tap-dancing around those issues, like why did you work for Bristol Myers for only 8 months. So I wasn't really ever blown away by any of them, although some of them were close to being hostile. They didn't last that way for long. There's always a definite distance there in the beginning, although some of them, the people were so friendly and we just sat down and talked. But by and large, they were fairly pleasant, fairly positive experiences.

Q:

Do you remember any specifics about your interviews? What were the different styles of interviews that you had?

A:

There were people that were very "give and take" in conversation. They'd really talk with you back and forth about things, and those were the best because you know how long to talk and how long not to talk. But if somebody's just sitting there quietly observing you, you struggle with thinking, "should I be talking a lot, saying everything I know about everything related to the topic or what?" It's a little bit more anxiety-producing. You're not getting any feed- back from the person or they're not talking with you, they're just listening. You have to be prepared for a little discomfort because you can't read the interviewer.

That's one of the courtesies when you're talking to somebody socially, is that you give them feedback, verbal or nonverbal. So the people that sat back and just sat there looking at you were kind of difficult, but they were few and far between. I would say that most of them were nice. There were maybe one or two of them who I would say were almost judgmental. It's easy to get anxious and preoccupied with, "how's this going, am I making sense?" Even for somebody who's been through a lot of interviews, although business interviews are never quite that stiff. Because they want to know what you're really like because they're going to work with you everyday. So they try to be themselves for you to see them, whereas some MD on the faculty could not give a rat's ass whether you like him or not. So that's how I think there's a big difference between the two.

Q:
Did you have other types of interviews at other places?

A:
Some had students interviewing. I had a couple of fourth years interview me.   One at SUNY at Syracuse I had a student interview me and I think that was good. And at University of Chicago I had a student interview me. Although they both said that they weren't really on the committee I didn't really become too loose with them either. You still want to sound buttoned-up a little bit. But as far as the format goes, just one-on-one almost always.

Q:
Do you remember any questions that you particularly liked or disliked?

A:
A lot of people asked, "so why are you going into medicine?" You start to sound like a broken record. You know, "why this change? You seem like you were doing well in business and marketing, why would you want to go into medicine?" It's a fair question, but you could turn that into something that you're either tired of talking about or you can use it as an opportunity to bring home everything you said in the personal statement and everything else. Even if you did a really good job of explaining it in your materials, it ought to be asked.   Especially if you're visibly not twenty-two which most of us aren't. We like to hope anyway. I hope I don't come across

as twenty-two.

Q:

So, how did you choose to go where you're going?

A:

Combination of all the things - location, the laid-back atmosphere or the non-cutthroat atmosphere. I wouldn't call it laid-back, but the notion that it wouldn't be this pressure cooker for four years. I wanted a school with a good reputation. My wife's family is from the Midwest. I didn't want to live in the Midwest frankly. My other choices were not any better in terms of reputation, so sort of the best of all of them.

Q:

So tell me, if you gave me your top few recommendations for non-traditional students from start to finish, from when you make the decision to when you get accepted, what would those be?

A:

Even before you're thinking of applying, you can get involved in some community activities and if they be medical or whether they just be community service type things, volunteering, being a Big Brother, being a volunteer counselor, whatever. It's good not only because it helps you get in, but it gets you into it and it gets you a little flavor of it. Some people may feel like they don't need that because they already know what they want to do, but what can it hurt? You're going to be eventually asked to do a million things at once and being able to do 10,000 things at once ahead of time is good. It's a skill and to demonstrate that you can, in my case, work 20 hours a week, 25 hours a week at night during the week, take all upper level courses and get a 4.0.

That's helpful for them to know that you can do that. And it's also good because it shows that you give a crap about the people side which you can definitely go overboard and sound like this warm and fuzzy person that everybody hates. But at the same time, it's helpful. So even before you do all that. When you're now taking your prerequisites whether it's the post-bacc program or not, don't let anything get in the way. Don't let your job if you're working during the day and doing this at night allow you to not do well because it's your last chance to show that you can do well, especially if you didn't excel as an undergrad. A lot of people don't. They can still be good doctors.

But the thing is that even when you're doing it, you know you're doing the right thing but there's no feedback. You're just out there for a year applying. You've done all your course work. Fortunately, I got a marketing job for that year and I was making a lot of money. And I knew that if I didn't get in, I could just stay here in New York City and love the East Village. That's where I was living — I had a great lag year, it was awesome. But doing the right things during the times when you're not getting a good sense of feedback or you don't really know how things are going to turn out, and yet being able to deal with that and just sort of live on the edge, not knowing for a long time if you will get into medical school. From the time that you decide to go back to school until the application year and then finally you start med school next Fall. And then even then, it takes you a while to sort of blend into the med school experience. So sort of keeping it in perspective while things are kind of stressful.

Q:
Is there anything else you want to add?

A:
Just that anything's possible and particularly if they didn't do well in school in undergrad. It's never never too late.

Q:
Thanks a lot.

Interview Nine — Susan Libman

SUSAN LIBMAN: Susan is thirty two and married. She graduated from Stanford with a degree in Political Science. After college, she worked in sales and marketing for a medical equipment company.

Q:
Tell me what you used to do before you made the decision to go to med school.

A:
I worked for a company called Medline Industries which is a Chicago-based company that manufactures medical and surgical products. And I worked for them for four years, two and one-half years I was a sales rep selling everything from Band-Aids to wheel-chairs out in California to hospitals and surgery centers. The last year and a half, I was a surgical specialist and I just sold surgical products, four basic surgical products.

But I didn't sell them directly — I helped sales reps sell them, so I traveled — I covered twelve states and I would travel with the sale reps in their territories helping them sell just these products I was responsible for. And the products were surgical instruments, surgical gloves, reusable surgical gowns made out of Gortex and sterile custom kits, like all the plastic basins and all the plastics and paper stuff that you use for a particular surgery. And so I did that for about a year and a half.

Q:
How about before that? In college, what was your original major?

A:
Well my major was political science.   I went to school thinking that I'd be premed because I've always been interested in medicine since I was in fifth grade when my teacher Mr. Putman made us learn all the bones in the body in fifth grade and several muscles — I knew the sternocleidomastoid in fifth grade. He totally turned me on to medicine. I was fascinated with the body as a machine. I was always more science and math oriented in high school and not English and history oriented.

In college I kind of got distracted and I felt that my track that I was on all of the sudden got much wider and filled with dif-ferent opportunities so I thought I would investigate other parts of myself that I didn't initially think I wanted to explore. So it could have been English, it could have been History, it could have been anything fuzzy I decided I wanted to do and try to improve my writing skills and analytical skills.   I wasn't as good in poli-sci as I was in science or in biology in high school by any means.   I was never — something was missing.

Q:
So when did you make the decision that in fact you wanted to go to medical school?

A:
It was four years after, when I was working for Medline. I felt like I didn't do medicine when everyone else was doing it or premed when everyone else was doing it, so it just seemed like I blocked it out as an option. That opportunity passed me and I just kept going forward and I really didn't stop and think about what would really make me happy.   So I went to go work for Medline, and they sent me back out to California which I was happy about — I knew I wanted to be there.   Luckily, the company I was working for was involved in medicine and that was a total coincidence. So I was exposed to surgery, all the ins and outs of a hospital, and clinicians.

And then finally what did it was a friend of mine. She was always science-oriented, she never did it, and she ended up going back. We were talking on the phone and we hadn't talked in six months, and she was telling me that she had just started med school at Penn. And she had taken 5 years off before going back, and she loved it. She put me in touch with other people who had gone back.

The more I could gather this information of people who had done it, I saw it was possible to do. Sure it had changed their lifestyle and yes, they were an older student and they knew how old they were going to be when they were done. All these things-that WAS the reason why I didn't go into it — all of the sudden I saw people coping with those things and dealing with them — and I thought, if they can do it so can I.

And then I realized there were all these programs. There were fifteen programs, these post-bacc programs. There was this network, this setup that made it possible when I thought that if you didn't do it your freshman or sophomore year of college, you couldn't do it. The more I gathered and could see it being done, I had no excuse not to do it. So I just quit my job and did it. And of course I took all my sciences over — it took me about two and a half years. I'm so happy I made that choice.

Q:
That's a huge decision. Obviously you had to go back and take more courses.

A:
Right. I took everything.

Q:
And where did you do that?

A:
I did probably 60% of it at Stanford. I took my biology and my chemistry there. I took my physics at a small community college outside, 10 miles outside Stanford, called Foothill Community College. Then I moved back to Chicago and finished up at DePaul and University of Chicago, biochemistry and organic chemistry lab. So I did it piecemeal everywhere.

Q:
So you took more than just the required premed courses?

A:
I took what was required for med schools and nothing more.

Q:
But you took biochemistry.

A:
Because I needed one additional organic chemistry quarter because Stanford only has two. And that qualified as organic chemistry. That's the only reason I took it, with a lab.

Q:
When you chose your courses, did you investigate the teachers or the courses?

A:
Yeah. The reason I decided to go to Stanford, despite the fact that it was really expensive to do it, was they have a premed advisor there. She put me in touch with people who had done this them-selves. I should take physics at Stanford, shouldn't I? Was it better to take it at Foothill? She networked for me and gave me all this information of people to contact so I could figure out what would be best for me. Yeah, it was very helpful. That was the reason why

I decided to go back there. I was thinking about doing it at a program like Bryn Mawr. I didn't do a program because I had to move outside of California. I needed support and to be around people who are going to support you.

Q:
Getting to your courses...When you studied, what did you use mostly for study aids? Did you use study groups and tutoring?

A:
I was really nervous when I first started. When I was in chemistry, I was in class with freshmen and in biology, I was in class with sophomores. I was thinking, I'm older, I should do better than these people. No excuse not to. So I was nervous. And I made a pact with myself that I would always prepare for class, I'd always do the reading before class and if I ever had questions, immediately after lecture, I would get them addressed then and there.

When I was an undergrad, I was more interested in getting out of lecture and going to meet my friends for lunch instead of mastering the material. I never went outside the boundaries of the class, I never pushed myself. I just didn't have the interest to do it. When I went back, I was so much more focused so I knew why I was there, that I was paying my money to be there, that I was going to make the most out of it. I wasn't going to let questions linger in my mind and figure them out later and never get to them. I really wanted to get on top of the material.

So I befriended the TA's really quickly and we'd end up having conversations about things. I'd go in with a couple of questions but they'd lead to other things and I'd read other materials. I bought books that weren't required for the class which I'd never done before and just found things at different angles. I befriended a couple of people in each of my classes, one or two people that became really strong study partners.

As far as doing things differently from undergrad, I think what I had in my favor was just bare interest in the material, much more than before. But as far as particular techniques, other than political science is completely different from studying science, I don't think I changed things that much. I used note cards which I do now. I made flash cards on things. That's how I study. I use flash cards so I compartmentalize what I know and what I don't know. Constantly testing myself.

Q:
So you did use some study groups?

A:
For biology and chemistry. Biology I studied with one person and chemistry, I studied with a different person. Physics I studied completely on my own, I wasn't in a group. It was a community college — there really wasn't a sense of community there. Everyone was living at home and commuting there. And most of those people had day jobs — it was a night class and so there really wasn't the time to get together.

Q:
You talked a little bit about your advisement. Did your advisor help you plan your class schedule and help you with your med school applications?

A:
Both.   At Stanford, they had a whole filing system on every medical school you can think of, and they have people write back after their first and second years on what they like about the school and what they don't like. So I'd read ones of the people who were postbaccs and then the advisor would suggest schools that liked postbacc people or schools that were easier to get into, schools that were stretches, schools that weren't stretches.   They have this whole relationship with all these different med schools too. If they make a phone call for you, it's a nice thing. They won't write recommendations for you, but they'll read your personal statement and tell you if it's good or if it's not. Or different essays, they'll help you with.

Q:
That's great. Tell me about your extra-curricular activities, during this time and from college on, both medical and non-medical?

A:
What did I do? I worked for the Disabilities Association, I TA'd the biology class that I took. My second year of taking classes, I TA'd that while I was taking classes and that was definitely a full-time job. Other than that, I played tennis tournaments and I took competitive tennis class at Stanford while I was there. Most of my activities were short-term.

I also worked at Stanford at the Center for AIDS Research. And it was a lab job - it was actual lab bench work. But I didn't like it at all. I also volunteered at San Francisco General Hospital in the emergency room which was once a week for about 5 hours. Very hands-on, you had to be CPR-certified. You were a patient advocate, you were in there in the trauma room, you were running around doing things for the nurses and the doctors, not just running to the lab to pick up paper. You were actually doing things. Talking to the patients when they're getting stitched, sutured. And then I also volunteered with a hospice program for people dying of AIDS . Also, I was in an AIDS buddy program. I think it was local to the San Francisco Bay area.

When I moved back to Chicago and took classes here, I worked at Evanston Hospital for a year. It was clinical research in the clinical pharmacology unit where they do drug testing.

Q:
Of all these things, what would you recommend if you were thinking not just of your own interests? What would you recommend to prospective students, as far as solidifying their interest or seeing if they're really interested and also, what would be good to help get into med school?

A:
I would do something clinical, do something very patient-oriented. And I'd do something research-oriented. Seeing as though those are two main paths you can take with medicine, and seeing which you're more comfortable in doing. On the research side, I would try to do clinical research and some bench science research and see if you have an interest in it. Before ruling something out, I would try it. I was always ruling out — I didn't want to go into research — but I'd never done it. So doing it reconfirmed my feelings, but I would do both if you could.

And definitely do something clinically-based where you're dealing with doctors and nurses and where you're having some patient contact so you get a feel for what it's like in the medical world as possibly a physician but also what it's like to treat sick people. I thought the AIDS Buddy program was great from a patient perspective. I would go grocery shopping for him and go over to his house and do things for him around the house and basically just be his friend.

Q:
So you had a lot of involvement. More than most people.

A:
Right, and I did not do it for a resume or whatever. I did it purely because I was interested in doing it. That was the ironic thing — when I did poli-sci, I wasn't interested in doing anything in politics

so I didn't do any volunteer stuff or get involved.

Q:
OK, moving on to MCAT. As far as spring or Fall, when did you take it and do you think it's important to take it one time or the other?

A:
I took it spring. I think it's much more important — I think you should take it in the spring rather than in the Fall. It took me two and a half years to do my premed stuff. There were friends of mine who did it in a year and a half. That's how most people did it. I just figured that I've waited this long, I can wait another year. Actually, I'm glad I did it, because I TA'd and I love teaching. I didn't have to study at all for biology for the MCATs because I taught it that year, and when you teach something, you learn it ten times better.

Q:
Did you take any review courses?

A:
I took Kaplan. I needed that structure, someone to force me to do it and for me to feel like I was getting a good review. Their study exams that they give, I don't think are really indicative of what's on the MCAT — they're much, much more difficult than what's on the MCAT and they're much more time-pressured than what's on the MCAT. Now in one sense that could be good because once you get to the MCAT, you feel good. But up to that point, when you're not doing well on those tests, you lose the confidence. If you go in knowing that, it might be more helpful. But the reason I took Kaplan was because I also took Kaplan for the GMAT and the LSAT, and so I got a discount.

Q:
So you organized your studying around Kaplan. How long did you study?

A:
Probably four months . That was plenty.

Q:
Now for the primary application, the AMCAS application, what did you feel was important in the non-essay part? What did you try and emphasize where you listed your activities?

Q:

I would say just showing diversity. Showing well-roundedness and I found it was important to put down leadership roles. Not just that I did this and did that, but that I led this and I organized that. And the things you were recognized for.   I had no academic awards so I had to rely more on things I accomplished in my job. I also really wanted to show how I exposed myself to different parts of medicine by doing the clinical stuff, doing the bench work, doing the patient stuff.   I wanted to expose myself to all those things.

Q:

That's really important. How about the essay? What did you write about?

A: I just wrote about how I came to the decision and how I got exposed to medicine. I was initially interested in medicine from a mechanical standpoint of how the body works, as a kid. I became interested in all the other aspects of care giving and the human side of medicine as I got older and matured. And I just walked through that progression of how my interest in medicine changed.

Another thing to really keep in mind though, is that I was told by many people who were post-baccs who were asked during their interviews, "Well, you've done all these things and you've tried all these different paths. What's to make us think that medicine isn't just another one of those paths and you're not going to change your mind?" So I think it's important to show that thread through your life of medicine, your interest in it, if that's you're story, if that's the truth. Show how you just aren't a spontaneous, frivolous kind of non-committal, that you don't have direction, that you're just bouncing off one career to the next. I think it's important to show how your story unfolds leading you towards medicine and why that's the right choice for you. I think that's important. They're going to be asking you that, they're going to be looking for that, and they'll be concerned about that. That's the one drawback I think about being a post-bacc.

Q:

How did you choose the schools which you applied to?

A:

I think I applied to 17 schools which was probably average. And I kept my California residency because I wanted to be in California. But then I had a big change in my life during this process of deciding where to go to med school, and meeting Andrew, my husband.

So my whole thing was to try to be in a place where he and I could work together and be happy together. And that led me a lot towards Chicago.

I applied to every school in Chicago except for Chicago Med. I always knew in the back of mind that it was going to be Northwestern, I have no idea how. Even before I ever interviewed or before I was granted an interview, I felt that was going to be where I ended up. I kept being told over and over - quality of life, be in a place where you're comfortable, meaning a city, in the part of the city. And Rush was not in a place I'd feel comfortable walking at night or a place where if I need to take a walk, I want to walk around that part of the city. Northwestern was right on the lake, it was in a great part of town, it was convenient, I could meet people, I had friends in this area. And I think I let that dictate more where I was going as opposed to what the particular school had to offer me.

Q:
How about other schools in the country?

A:
I applied to all the California schools except for a couple, and I did not apply anywhere East except for University of Vermont because one of my best friends from my post-bacc program is actually there now. And we wanted to go to school together. And that's it, mostly. There's some here and there, I liked St. Louis and stuff. Otherwise, Chicago and California were the big ones.

Q:
How about your secondary applications? What was your general impression of the different ones that you had? How did you try to use the secondary application?

A:
I did everything just by the books. What they asked for, I gave. I don't think I did a lot of sending extra letters of recommendation, although I did for Northwestern. I sent an extra one from a guy I worked for at Northwestern, which I think helped a lot.

I really wanted to get in to San Francisco, UCSF. I had the head charge nurse at San Francisco General emergency room write me a letter of recommendation for my volunteering there, and I wrote several letters there telling them how they were my first choice. I never got in there to get an interview there. So other than

that, I went by the books. I answered questions the way they wanted. I didn't send videotapes or send tapes or do anything different
except for those things I mentioned.

And the other thing I did was the way I prepared my
essays. I did it all on computer and then I went to Kinko's and printed it out and pasted it on it. I was to the margin on every single
essay. I did the font — I would print things over and over until
they'd fit the space exactly. It was kind of messy and I used a glue
stick. Sometimes I'd look at it and go, god, it doesn't fold right.
After a while, you just send it.

And I made copies of everything. I had a file for each
school. I'd write a checklist because each folder would need different things.   And I would have the deadline or whatever the due
date was, and each time I'd add things that were needed to the file,
I would check it off and when everything was checked, I'd put it in
and send it out. I also had a calendar that had each one's due date
on it. So I never missed a deadline, never missed a letter of recommendation.

The other thing about letter of recommendations was at
Stanford, they have a file where you could keep everything confi-
dential on file there, and then when you want something sent out,
you write to them or you fax to them what school and what letters,
and they send them directly from there. So I never touched those,
but you have to follow up to see if those get there because a couple of mine didn't.

Q:
That happened to me. Eight schools never got them.

A:
Always follow up on letters of recommendation . Follow up with
professors to make sure they've submitted it to your file. Check
with the professor to make sure they've submitted the file to wherever you kept everything and follow up with the schools to make
sure they got them. If you want, also follow up with the place that's
holding your file to make sure they've sent what they said they
were going to, all those things. It's a full-time job — I mean we
should get paid for it!

Q:
You talked about your recommendations a lot.   How did you
choose who you wanted to write them for you?

A:
They were people who knew me very well, not necessarily people that held big positions. And that's key — that was what I was advised to do. Even though someone is the president of some company that you worked for, if they don't know who you are, they aren't going to write you an outstanding recommendation. It's going to be generic; it's not going to stand out. For me, at our age, it was very easy to get letters of recommendation because we could have that rapport with people that we worked for or worked with. Also, because I befriended professors and I was a TA, and even in the classes I wasn't a TA I knew my professors pretty well.

Q:
So you'd recommend to really try to get to know your professors. Besides getting your questions answered, you'd know them well enough to give you a recommendation.

A:
You shouldn't just ask for the recommendation from someone you got the A in their class. Because all they'll write is that you got an A — your transcript shows that. You need to find someone who knows you and your motivations and your study habits and your interest and the way you work. That's much more important than getting the department head to write you something generic. The other thing you probably should ask the professor before they write it is, can you write me a positive recommendation? Because I've heard of people that will write a recommendation that is not a good one. They should turn it down and say they won't write it. They should say let's find someone else to write you one because I can't do it, but make sure the people you're asking are writing good recommendations.

A friend of mine, he was an undergrad. He was Phi Beta Kappa, he was an RA. He was doing an honor's project, science biology project, with a big head honcho guy at Stanford. Halfway through the honor's project, he decided not to do it and really pissed off this guy who I guess had invested a lot of time in him. And for some reason, he asked him to write him a recommendation and the guy agreed to do it, but he wrote a scathing one. My friend didn't get into any school, not even his safety schools. And so with one of his safeties, he called them and he said, "Can you tell me why I didn't get in. I know that sounds odd, but I just don't understand. All my numbers are way above your averages." And they told him that it was that letter of recommendation. Luckily Yale called him and said, "We've lost your letters of recommendations, will you resend them?" He resent them minus that one. That's the only place he got in, and that's where he went.

Q:
Did you update your application?

A:
Yes. I took a biochemistry class. Right, I sent out a letter. But transcript-wise, I was still taking biochemistry while I was applying to school, so I sent that. I may have sent an extra letter of recommendation from the guy I worked for at the hospital in Evanston. I think I sent letters to a number of schools. Also, If there's a way you can make yourself stand out by either going to that school and meeting with someone or talking to someone, I would do it. Because people get in for strange reasons.

Q:
As far as your interviews went, I guess there are different areas I wanted to cover - what questions they asked, how you chose which ones to go to, and the different types from individual to panel?

A:
I wore a suit. I basically went to every interview I got, except for Vermont. All my interviews were on-on-one except for Northwestern. University of California Davis held my interview during their winter break so no one was there. I never got a tour, I never met a student. And so if you get one, make sure it's not over a break or ask to come at a different time if you can. I think you need to get a feel, as best as you can, for the atmosphere at that school. Sit in on a class. I did that at Loyola. And also at University of California Davis, they had this guy who had only been with them for a month interview me. He could tell me more about Harvard than he could tell me about Davis. But he was my favorite guy there, which says a lot about that school. So that didn't help me very much in getting a feel for that school.

Northwestern was a panel and I didn't like it, so of course I came here. Loyola was the warmest, most friendly. Everyone there really wanted you to feel comfortable. They wanted you to go there, you got that sense. Maybe a little too much. Rush's interviews were probably the most formal. But I'd say for the most part, they didn't have a set number of questions, they didn't ask me tricky questions. They just wanted to know who I was, get a feel for who I was. And that's the type of place I'd like to go to anyhow.

Although I have to say to take your interview with a grain

of salt in giving you a sense of what the school's like because it's a totally different part of the school. The administration and the admissions office are not people you're going to encounter everyday when you're in med school. So if while you're at that school, if you have an opportunity to sit in class or really meet a professor or go to the hospital or meet students, you need to do that.

You can only get so much out of an interview. And in fact, my interview at Northwestern was the worst interview of all of them. From my side. I didn't like it. The five other students interviewing that day were from Johns Hopkins and they were a most intense, cutthroat group, it was horrible!

And I talked to one of the Deans. The one thing I did like about Northwestern was that they didn't cut down other schools in Chicago.

Q:
Do you remember any specific questions that were interesting?

A:
I had one guy ask me, gave me a hypothetical: if I have my one year old daughter and it was her birthday and my beeper went off and I had an emergency, what would I do? Which I doubt he would have asked a man, but he asked me. I answered the question, but I thought it was an inappropriate question.

Other than that, people basically wanted to know why I wanted to be in med school. Or they'd give me hypotheticals. And the hypotheticals were to give them a sense of how I work through problems, what my thought processes are, not whether I answered it right or if I was going to do the right thing, or if that's what doctors should do. It was more they wanted me to verbalize what I would think about.

At Northwestern, I was given a hypothetical — I'm an allergist and a ten year old patient comes in with his mom, and he's been my patient for years and mom's had a drug problem, but she went to rehab. But during this appointment, she leaves the room and goes to the bathroom and she's in the bathroom for 15 seconds and she comes back, and she's in a completely altered mood — what do you do? I had no idea what I'd do, but I spoke about what I'd be thinking and what my next steps might be, but I didn't know what I was legally able to do. I knew what my priorities were, and they wanted to know my priority is my patient. I need to take care of my patient, but his mother does too, and he's going to go home with his mother, and is that the best thing for him? How can I detain them, who do I call, would I call someone or try to handle it on my own? Those are the things they want to know. How you think about difficult situations.

Q:
Thanks.

Interview Ten - Allison Mangurten

ALLISON MANGURTEN: Allison is a twenty-seven years old. She graduated from the University of Illinois, Champaign-Urbana, with a degree in Business Administration. After college, she worked as a CPA for a public accounting firm.

A:
My name is Allison Mangurten and I am 27.

Q:
What did you do before coming to medical school?

A:
Before I came to med school I was an accountant. I worked for a little bit over two years for a public accounting firm and after that I went back to school for a year to take science which I had never even heard of. Then I applied to med school for a year and during that year I worked in a lab and did research.

Q:
Tell me about your decision to go back to medical school.

A:
I thought when I went to college that I was going to be premed and I was just taking the general requirements for everything. And then I decided that I really didn't want to be in school that long so I started thinking that business classes would be interesting. I thought accounting could be a good career because I was good at math and it was really easy at that time — well it still is — to get a job and get paid really well and you get great benefits. But the reason it's so easy to get a job is because the jobs stink, so people leave. I really didn't stop to think about that when I was in college. So I started working and I hated it and I thought about every career in the world from being a travel agent to being an aerobics instructor — I was going to open my own aerobics studio. And then I realized what I was trying to avoid was going back to school which is what I really did want to do. So I started researching what I exactly had to do to apply to med school and the whole process took me about two years. It just took me two years to decide that I was going to quit. My parents wouldn't let me quit without a plan - I couldn't just quit and hang out . I had to have a plan.

Q:
So you had a plan. And you needed to take premed courses?

A:
Right I had to take all of them. I mean I had never taken any of them, so I took a science crash course for a year.

Q:
Did you go through a specific program?

A:
I went to Loyola. They market their program as a post-bacc science program so that was what I originally heard about when I started asking questions to people.   It turns out that it's really just classes. We're integrated with all the other undergrads — It's not like you're in a separate program. So the advantage to going there is probably that you get priority registration, which is good for people who are trying to work part-time. If you only have specific hours that you can take classes, it's real easy to get classes because they let you register first and then the undergrads get to register.   I also looked into going to U of Illinois.   The classes are the same basically — basic biology, chemistry, organic, physics— but it's really hard to get into classes at U of I because you get last priority registration. You have no hours and you're not getting a degree so they don't really care. Most people I talked to that went there- it was taking them 2 to 3 years to finish their post bacc. classes because they couldn't get in. And I knew I wanted to do it in a year and I knew it shouldn't take that long so — I mean I was basically trying to avoid the tuition at Loyola. But in light of the tuition I'm paying now, it's really not that big of deal.

Q:
So you took the basic year of biology, year of physics, chemistry, organic. Did you take any extra classes?

A:
No. I took the minimum you could take to get in.

Q:
Did you go about any special methods of choosing your courses or teachers for your pre med courses?

A:
A little bit, but I was more concerned with the times of the classes

because I worked part-time for a little bit. I worked during tax season at my old job. It was nice to be able to come back and work on my old clients. So I took classes in the morning and would go to work in the afternoon. I was limited to whoever was teaching at that time. Some of the teachers - if there were two at the same time - I would try to find out about the better one. People have different opinions though, and it's always hard to tell.

Q:
Since you worked part-time, how many courses did you take at a time?

A:
I think I took three and the lab. Well three classes and then two labs. It was pretty crazy! I went to school in the morning, went to work in the afternoon and studied at night. It was nuts. I think I started in May and I took just general chemistry over the summer and the lab. And then in the fall, I took organic, physics and bio and then the organic and the biology lab. And then I did the second part of all of that in the spring. So I never actually finished the physics lab. I just took half of it over the next summer and then I got into Northwestern and they don't require you to take it. So I dropped out of the second semester. Opted out of electricity.

Q:
When you were studying, what different types of study aids did you use? Did you use your notes from class, did you use old notes, did you get a hold of old tests, did you use study groups, did you use tutoring?

A:
Mostly my notes and the books for the classes. I just used my notes. They don't really have old tests available. They didn't really have old notes or a note service so basically just my own notes and books. Divine inspiration. It just all came to me in a flash.

Q:
Did you use a school advisor?

A:
I went to see the Director of the Loyola program before I started and he tried to discourage me from going to med school. He told me I'd never get in, that there were too many doctors. He gave me all the statistics about the people applying and how few got in and it

was so impossible. It got me really upset when I was in there. I thought, "You don't know anything about me. You haven't seen my transcript and you don't know one thing other than that I was an accountant." So I was really upset and I didn't want to go to school there almost because of it. But then I realized I was not going to interact with him everyday.

I asked him about it later, having met with him because you have to meet with him later to get a letter of recommendation. I said, "Do you do that to everybody or was that just for my benefit?" He basically said that he just wants to make sure that the people in the program were really serious. He wants you to make an informed decision. So that was his big thing — informed consent — that he was just telling it like it was. Maybe he does scare off some people that really shouldn't be there. But they were really good about deadlines, sending out our recommendations and advising us where we should apply. It was pretty good. I think actually he's left since then. I heard he left.

Q:
So they did help you with application process?

A:
Yeah. They sent out all the recommendations and they kept files on everybody. They were usually pretty timely. They had a lot to do and they were pretty good about it.

Q:
And they helped you decide where to apply?

A:
Not really. I figured no one really knows how people get into med school. It's a big mystery, so I just guessed a little bit. I didn't apply to Harvard - I thought that would be a waste of my $50.

Q:
So where did you apply?

A:
I applied to all the schools in Chicago. I guess there's six of them. Then I applied to Wash U. I applied to University of Michigan, and I applied to UCSF which I'm sure they just couldn't wait to throw out my application. Great, we don't have to look at this one. Actually I sent my first applications to more places than that. My first one I sent to Georgetown. I sent one to somewhere in

Pennsylvania. Wisconsin. Well I stayed pretty much Midwest. The Big Ten. I really had no idea. I was picking schools that I had heard of. My dad gave me a couple of recommendations of places that he heard of and that he knew people who had gone there. I thought I wanted to stay in Chicago just because I thought it would be my best chance of getting in being a resident. But I wish I had better help knowing where to apply because I just guessed.

Q:
How about extracurricular activities?   What did you participate in before you came to school?

A:
I volunteered at Children's Memorial Hospital for a while. They have a fund raising board that raises money for the hospital and for various research things. So I worked on that a little bit. I did research for a year at Northwestern in a lab here. But I worked in microbiology, never even walked in a lab before. Walked in the first day, I thought my boss was going to pass out — Okay, what's a pipette? She's saying to herself, "How am I ever going to train this girl?" She trained me, she was great. She taught me everything.

Q:
You did her taxes.

A:
It worked out great. I really thought it was interesting. I really wanted to learn so she didn't mind teaching me because I tried really hard. I wanted to be there. I think most people don't mind helping you if you show you're trying. I played extracurricular volleyball and softball.   It's not really medically related.

Q:
That's good. Do you think your research experience helped you get in?

A:
Probably. Not necessarily the research per se but the fact that I knew some people here. I'd been around the university. I had recommendations from my boss who is on the medical school faculty. One of the doctors I worked with made some calls for me, actually to describe me to the Dean. So I don't know. They say they can't do that much if you don't get in otherwise, but they can highlight your name. So I think that helped.

Q:
So if you're giving people advice, would you say to seek out opportunities like that?

A:
Yeah, it can't hurt you. I think if you're definitely underqualified, you could have the President of the United States call and I don't know if that would help. But if you're qualified and you get someone who knows someone who can call for you, it can't hurt. If nothing else, at least when you go into the interview, they put your face with the name. A lot of times people who are completely qualified don't get in because they slip through the cracks somehow. I think whatever you can do to make sure you don't, more power to you I say. You know what they say — it's not what you know in life, it's who you know. Unfortunately there's a lot of truth to it.

Q:
Definitely. How about the MCAT? Tell me about your MCAT experience. When do you think people should take it?

A:
I took it in the spring. Everyone told me if I waited it would ruin my chances. By the time they get your application, they've already accepted everybody. I took it in the spring. I probably didn't go about the process in the best way. I didn't take a review class which I probably should have. I've only taken one other review class ever in my life before for the CPA, and I went the first day and I never went back. I paid for the class, I got all the notes from it, but I never once went after the first day. I just don't learn well in class situations. I need to just sit down with the books and just study. So I figured instead of wasting six hours a week sitting in this room, having someone talk to me about the CPA, I'd rather sit and study the material. So I used the same rationale for the MCAT.

I got the Flowers MCAT review. I basically studied out of that, I did a lot of old tests. I sent away for the practice ones. Did a lot of those - I think those are really good. And you know at the time, I was still taking classes. I was finishing my spring semester classes at the same time. I was still learning new material right up until the test. In retrospect, I might have taken a review class. Just because I think that in the classes, they highlight the really important things. I don't know if it would have affected my score at all, but it might have been worth my time.

Q:
How did you organize your studying?

A:
The book that I had (Flowers) broke it down by section. I just went through each section.   I just studied the important concepts and I did make note cards on the important formulas. That's basically the week right before, that's what I studied off of, the note cards. Just to make sure I knew the formulas that I thought would be important and did a couple of more practice tests.   I think the biggest thing is the timing. I think that if I had all day to take the MCAT I could get a perfect score. But I think the timing is a much bigger factor than I realized, and I think that's where a review class would help you. Just to get you used to the timing. I timed myself, but it's a lot easier to cheat when you're sitting at home in your kitchen than when you're in a test situation. I think that was my biggest problem was running out of time when I actually took the test.

Q:
And how many months did you study for?

A:
The test was in April. I pretended to start in January, flipping through the review book. I probably went through the review book twice. I didn't get really serious about it probably until the month before. And even then, I was having problems really focusing because I just had so much else going on too. I was taking classes and I was still working a little. I should have probably bagged the working, in retrospect.

    To be honest, I didn't do that great on the test. I was debating about taking it again when I got my score. And I didn't know what to do. I called every admissions person in the city of Chicago and asked what I should do. I literally got a 50-50 response. Half the people told me just to apply, it's better to get your application in early. I had really good grades and a really mediocre MCAT score. And my big question was, do these compensate for each other? They'll look at my grades say, "oh, this girl is a genius." And then they'll look at my scores and say, "Okay, this girl doesn't know how to read!" Half the people said take it again and half the people said just apply. I just didn't want to take the test again. I just decided to send everything in and kind of prayed. And I got lucky.

Q:
How about the AMCAS application? Start with the non-essay part

that was mostly just information. What did you try to highlight on yours?

A:
I probably tried to highlight my grades the most. They were really good, consistently all the way through college and through the post-bacc classes. I put in all my extracurriculars from college and after college just because I think the more information you put on there, maybe something on there will catch someone's eye that really interests them. My dad interviews people for residencies and he'll come home and say, I met the greatest guy, he gardens just like I do! I'm saying, "Dad, what does that have to do with medicine?" Well it's the common interest.

Probably the more information you put down that shows that you're well rounded is better. So, I highlighted probably my grades and then my work experience because I thought that was kind of different. If nothing else, they could say "that's the one that's the accountant." Anything to make yourself stand out when you think these people are reading billions of applications stacked up on the desk.

Q:
Okay, how about your essay? What did you write about?

A:
My essay. I wrote about - I remember I wrote it a million times too - I wrote about why I left accounting to go to med school, and I remember the hardest thing for me was trying to make it sound like a positive change.   I didn't want to make it sound like I hated accounting and that's why I'm going to med school, because I thought that people would think well maybe she'll hate med school and she'll quit that and do something else. Just the wording of it was really hard, trying to say that I like this, but I think there's something more that I can do — there's something else. I think that's a really important thing if you're leaving a career to make it sound like it was okay, it wasn't terrible, but you think that med school interests you more. I don't think people want to hear anything negative about why you left. That's the hardest thing in the interview too, not make it come out negative. I think that's key if you're leaving a career because you don't want people to think that you can't commit and stay in a job, especially if you've had multiple jobs. If you've had three or four different careers, what's to say you're going to finish med school.

I had a really creative analogy that I drew in my essay that tied the whole thing together. I started out with a quote and tied the quote into this whole reason why I left and concluded by referring to the quote. The quote was kind of different. It was from this book The Tao of Pooh . It explains the theory of Tao according to Winnie the Pooh. The quote talked about how if you added up all the times in your life where you're at your goal versus if you add up all the times in your life where you getting to your goal, the times you spend getting there so far outweigh the times when you're actually there, so you have to enjoy the process. Basically that's it — you have to enjoy the process of getting to your achievement, not just the achievement itself or you'll be miserable. So I talked about how I didn't enjoy the process of being an accountant and how I thought I'd enjoy the process of med school. Somehow it tied all together. I know that's probably how I got an interview at U of C. Because it was kind of a cerebral thing that I wrote.

I think you do have to explain why you left your previous career path. I think to just apply and say that I've always wanted to be a doctor — well then why didn't you do it right away? You can't just leave those questions unanswered.

I'm not a writer at all. Then the problem too is that when you write these essays and you give them to various people to read, and everyone who reads it has a different opinion. My dad read it and he said, well you can take out this paragraph. He had a friend on some admissions committee — he read it and said well you definitely need to add in this. Plus they only give you a page so you really ought to pick and choose what you want on there. If you use six point font so they won't be able to read it they'll throw it out. I guess you gotta go with whose opinion you trust the most or whose you think is the most valid.

Q:
Obviously you had a number of secondary applications to fill out. Do you remember any essay questions that you thought were good and how you used those to your advantage?

A:
I actually really liked the application for Rush. It was partly annoying — it was really really detailed — but I thought the questions really asked you a lot and I thought they could really learn a lot about you from the questions. And I liked them too because they were short answers. It was questions like what are your strengths, what are your weaknesses and kind of interview-type questions. Like who would be your big support — personal support, I think, during med school.

Q:
Who did you say for that?

A:
I think I said my family because they live in Chicago. There was one question on the U of C application that was really offending when I read it. It was a very snobby question. I think it was the last question on there and I was very offended when I read it, so I wrote a really sarcastic answer back because I didn't really want to go there anyway and didn't care that much. That and my AMCAS essay are why I got an interview. I think they thought, oh this girl's a free thinker, she's not just going to agree — I mean I completely contradicted whatever their question was. I said I think this is wrong and this is why.

Northwestern asked about their new curriculum, if you knew about it, why you thought you could benefit from it. And I think I used that because I worked at Northwestern so I interacted with a lot of people, and I knew a lot about the curriculum and I did think I would work well in a curriculum like this versus more structured, more traditional. So I think I played that the right way.

Q:
Did you update your application after your secondary? Did you send in extra material?

A:
I did. In the lab I was working at, we were publishing a paper so I just sent a quick note to all the schools I was still interviewing at, just for their information, this is more of what I'm doing, just to show that I'm still interested and that I'm still trying if nothing else. I don't know if it necessarily matters all that much what you're sending in to places, as that you are . But any little thing I think to get your file on their desk again is important.

During the interview at Northwestern, they tell you that if you don't get in right away you could come and bug them every-day. I remember thinking the day of the interview that I work here. I was like, cool, I could just stop on the way to lab, and ask where's my application? I could come in at lunch, handcuff myself to the chair. It shows that you're really motivated. I think coming back from working too, you understand how to play some of those games.

Q:
Did you apply early?

A:

I think I postmarked my AMCAS application the day that they first started accepting them to the post office.

Q:

Tell me about the different schools that you applied to. Did you apply to a range of schools?

A:

I kind of thought that U of Illinois would be a safety for me, which it turns out that it wasn't. U of I's a state school. They just take your scores and your grades and just match it up. If you fall in the in box, you're in. If you fall in the out box, you're not. My score was so low that I got on the wait list. And there's so many applications, I didn't really know what a safety school was — I don't think there are any more. People had told me that Chicago Med was a safety school. I applied there and when I was at the interview day, they were telling us their statistics — they get more applications than any other school for some reason.

Q:

How did you choose the people for your recommendations?

A:

The people who I had the best rapport with, who I felt knew me the best and could write the best recommendation. Some teachers are just more creative, and they care more about the students. There were some teachers that I would go to their office hours more than others. I just felt they knew me on a personal level more than just, oh, she got an A in my class.

Q:

And then you had your research. Did you send a letter from the doctor you worked with?

A:

I think that is the other thing I sent in later. When I sent the article we had published, I sent her recommendation along with it. I didn't get it at first because I didn't know her well enough. I started my job right as I was sending out my applications. I didn't really think she would have anything to say about me. I didn't want it to come across fake. If I had asked her, I'm sure she would have written something. But I wanted it to be genuine. So I waited and then even after I sent in my secondaries, I sent in a supplemental recommendation from her. By then, she knew me well enough. I did-n't even think I thought about it, but she said, well I can write you something for here if you want. Then I thought, well if she's going to do that I might as well send it everywhere. So that's how I did it. I think I also had an employer, my old manager for my job. He wrote me a recommendation. And I had one from U of I in Champaign from a teacher that I had a really good relationship with there. So I just figured that diversity — not to have all my rec-ommendations from one place.   Just to show consistency.

Q:
So you had a lot of recommendations.

A:
I think I maybe had three or four originally and then I sent in extra. Well Loyola also, they keep a file on you and they send out all your recommendations. So they won't let you pick and choose. I had two or three teachers at Loyola who wrote me recommendations and then I had one from U of I and one from my old manager all in a folder together. So if you tell them to send your recommen-dations somewhere, they send all or none. If I had been doing it myself, I probably would have not included all of them to every place. Because I think you can probably overkill, send in like 20 recommendations. Admissions committee members then might ask , what's wrong with this person that they need half the world to write something for them. But it's probably good if you're applying as a non-traditional student, to get recommendations from different places just to show consistency. From undergraduate, to your job, to your post bacc. The longer you can show that you're a cool per-son for, the better it is for you I would think.

Q:
I think that's true. Tell me about your interviews.

A:
I only went to three. Questions that they asked me, except for here, are pretty much what you'd think. Like why'd you leave accounting. If you're leaving a profession, you've got to have a really good way to explain it because everyone's going to ask you that. It's the obvious question to ask. I think places asked me what I liked about my job before. At U of C they asked me a lot about my research. So if you put something on your application, you bet-ter be able to support it because they'll pick it out and try to find out if you just have something on there to fluff it up.

        If you put an extracurricular activity on there, you'd better
have done it because I think people are going to read through it.
Or at least be able to say something about it; don't just put it down.
They asked me a lot about my research and in a lot more detail
than I had expected. I could talk about it, I was doing it, but I did-
n't practice as much because I didn't think they'd get that detailed.
It depends on who's interviewing you too. If you get some clinician
interviewing you, they probably aren't going to ask you as much
about molecular biology as a Ph.D.

        My interview at Northwestern was really fun. I had a great
time. The panel interview part. I think it worked to my advantage
because the other two people did not interview well. One of the
two people offended one of the interviewers during the interview,
and the other person could barely speak English. So between the
two of them, I looked acceptable. It was relative to who is in your
panel. Hopefully you think you're not getting compared to the
other two people, but you can't help but compare. It's human
nature. One guy totally offended the interviewer.

Q:
What did he do?

A:
He didn't mean to, and I totally saw how it happened. They were
asking him about what specialty did he see himself going into, what
would be his focus? And he was trying to answer primary care. So
he's saying something like, "I really don't think I want to go into
anything high powered, just something like primary care." The
way it came out totally minimized primary care. Then he continued saying, maybe something like pediatrics and one of the interviewers was a pediatrician. The way he said it just made it sound
like any idiot off the street could be a pediatrician. I don't even
think he realized he did that. So I'm sitting there saying oh my god,
he just totally offended her....I was watching her, I was watching the
pediatrician's face and you could tell she was offended. And he
just went on, not realizing that he shouldn't have said that. He's
not in our class now.

        Also, we had to do some group activity. We had to write
things on the board as a group, generate a list. It was almost like
problem based learning type scenario, not medical. But we had to
put a bunch of characteristics on the board. I guess just to see if you
can work in a group. I remember one interviewer asking me a
question trying to see if he could make me change my mind. He
said would you ever be in a situation where you would deny some-

body care. And I said well I can't think of any specific situation, no, possibly there's one out there, but no, I think if I'm trained to treat someone and I'm capable of it, no. He says, what if someone comes to your office and demands an antibiotic? I answered "do they need one?" And he said no. Then I said "I wouldn't give it to them." Then he said, "well, isn't that denying care?" He was trying to get me to trip up. I said "no, it may be denying the care they want but that doesn't mean you're denying them care. If they came in demanding heart surgery and nothing was wrong with their heart, am I going to operate on them? No. It depends on your definition of care." We got into this discussion. He kept on me. Finally I said "I'm not going to agree with you, I'm sorry." I think I said, "look, I'm not going to define care that way." I didn't say it in a mean or rude way. I think they try to see if you'll change your opinion, if you'll back down or if you can make up your mind.

The other thing that worked to my advantage was one of the people who interviewed us...he retired this year I think...but he had gone to Kellogg and he had gotten an MBA. He was something in the med school, the Dean of something, but more the business aspect of it. I could talk to him at the business level because I had a business degree, and I think that helped me out. And my dad was a pediatrician so the pediatrician liked me.

Q:
Did you bring that up at all?

A:
I think she actually brought it up. I think she recognized my name and asked me afterwards, not during the interview. She's asked, "is this your dad?" It ended up that she knew him or she knew of him.

Maybe you go into the physicians' kids file. I wouldn't avoid it. If someone asked me directly, I would say yes. But I didn't make a point of bringing it up because I don't know if it'll help you or not, it depends. Some people might think it's great, oh, you know what it's like, you've seen it firsthand. But some people might say it doesn't matter.

Q:
What did you wear to your interview?

A:
I wore a suit, but it was an off-red color. I remember thinking specifically about what I should wear. I had a closet full of suits and most of them are black or dark. I was concerned about the

style and the color. It still was more like making yourself stand out. When I walked in, every person was wearing a black or blue suit, white shirt. I figured when they were talking about me later, they'll be like Okay, she's the one in the red suit.

Just to show that you're an individual I think. It depends too where you're going. I think you should definitely wear a suit because you're going to an interview. Make yourself stand out, like wear a scarf — wear something, but you gotta show that you respect the idea of an interview. That's why you should wear a suit.

Q:
Are there any general recommendations that you'd want to pass on?

A:
I guess probably just be yourself. I don't think you can make your-self something you're not. You can try — you can put all this stuff down on your application. You can try to fake it in the interview, but I think they'll see that — I mean a good interviewer will see it. Maybe you can fool some people but if it's not genuine, they'll see through it.

I guess the best thing is just to be confident. The whole process, I think, is just out there to ruin your confidence. You just gotta somehow believe that you're going to get in somewhere and just try. It can't hurt to send your application anywhere and every-where. Because it's not what you would think- where you would think the state schools and the less big-name schools are easier to get into. I don't think that's necessarily true. I think the better places that have a better reputation take more diverse students. They don't look for the cookie-cutter — this MCAT score, this grade, and that's it — and that helped me. It wouldn't have helped someone else maybe, but you just have to try.

Interview Eleven - William McCullough

WILLIAM MCCULLOUGH: Bill is married and thirty-one years old. His undergraduate degree is in Computer Science from Purdue University . Before coming to medical school, he spent eight years in the U.S. Navy as a line officer. He also has Master's in Business Administration.

A:
My name is William McCullough and my age is thirty-one.

Q:
What you did before you came to medical school?

A:
My undergraduate degree is in computer science. Before coming to medical school, I spent eight years in the U.S. Navy as a line officer. I spent two years in flight school and spent three years flying with a squadron both in the U.S. and overseas. I spent three years after that as an ROTC instructor.

Q:
How did you go about making your decision to go back to medical school? What led you up to that point?

A:
I had joined the Navy to fly and I was in a squadron flying, and came to the realization that there was not much of a future in doing what I was doing. I used to chase Soviet submarines. They don't come out as much as they used to, so the future of doing what I was trained to do in the Navy didn't look so good. So I started to consider other alternatives. Medicine was something that I was thinking about while I was in high school. Something that my mother, who was a nurse, kind of discouraged. And flying was something that my father was enthusiastically supportive of, so that is why I ended up flying initially. After realizing that there was not a long term future in it I made the decision to pursue medicine.

Q:
Being in the military, did they give you any sort of encouragement or did you seek advice from your commander?

A:
When I was in the squadron we had a flight surgeon, a navy doctor that is trained in aviation medicine assigned to us and I spent a lot of time with my flight surgeon talking about medicine. He was very encouraging. When I took the job at the ROTC that kind of was a career ender in the flying Navy. You need to stay flying if you are going to continually progress. So I took that with the full intention of pursuing an advanced degree and preparing for medical school. My commander at that ROTC unit was very supportive of my pursuit of a masters degree (MBA) and my pursuit of a medical career. And he even more supportive when I told him that I decided to take a Navy scholarship and stay in the navy after medical school as a navy doctor.

My masters is in business and administration from Virginia Tech. It was kind of a fall back if the medical school thing did not work out. I had intended to get out of the Navy and what I was going to fall back on was my computer education.

Q:
Did you take your masters courses while you were still in the Navy?

A:
Yes, while I was teaching and taking medical school prerequisites, I took the MBA course. I was essentially a full time student and working full time for three years.

Q:
Tell me about your premed courses and how you chose the ones you took and where you took them.

A:
I took calculus based physics as an undergraduate student at Purdue because the Navy requires that every officer that is going through an ROTC program takes calculus based physics. I took one semester of chemistry there as well just to fulfill a science elective. When I went back to Virginia Tech to teach and to take course work I had very limited time between my master's program and the twenty semester credit hours of science courses just to fulfill the basic prerequisites. I was kind of pressed.

At Virginia Tech I took the biology sequence. One year of biology. I took second semester chemistry and took organic chemistry both semesters. I was fortunate to convince the MBA program to allow me to take two electives outside of the school of business and because my professional goal was medicine, they allowed me to do that. I was able to take an undergraduate histology course, which was an excellent course. I also was able to take a graduate level neurochemical control course, which was pretty good.

Q:
Did your extra courses come in handy at medical school?

A:
It did help with the biochemistry of the neurotransmitters although we just brushed on it in the CNS course. Having had that in detail was very helpful. I wish I had taken a biochemistry course. I had an advisor at Virginia Tech, a biology professor who volunteered to be my advisor because no one in the MBA program could advise me as far as medical school goes. And she recommended biochemistry and histology course because this histology course was so good at Virginia Tech. Unfortunately, I could not take the biochemistry course, I just did not have the time for it.

Q:
Did you put in any effort into investigating the different teacher possibilities for each premedical course?

A:
Oh, sure. Every step of the way. Not really my first semester there because I was new. I didn't know anyone, I did not have any contacts. But I did it both with the MBA program and with the hard science prerequisites. Once I had a professor that I knew well, that knew me well as a student, I would seek their advice and seeing who was teaching the different classes that were offered and who would be the best person to take the course from.

Q:
When you were studying, what different materials did you use to study from? Books, old notes , old tests, your notes?

A:
Primarily textbooks. I am an adamant textbook reader. I read my textbooks before going to lecture to gain a foundation, the background, so I understand what's going on in lecture. That was always very helpful. I found that very few students read the textbook. In premed, very few students would do all assigned work or other problems that were not assigned, and that they weren't getting a grade for. For example, a recommended chemistry or organic chemistry question set- if they were not being collected or grad-

ed many students would not do them. Some students would do a few of them. I always did all of them. Additionally, any time a professor offered a help session, I went to the help session regardless of how I was doing in the course. Help sessions that professors offer are not just for the students that are struggling. They are for any student who has any question. I found it very helpful to take organized questions to help sessions and get all my questions answered before going into any exam rather than getting them all answered after going into an exam.

Q:
Did you use study groups or did you study by yourself?

A:
I did use study groups- not initially and not so much through the biology courses, but for chemistry, organic, histology and neuro-chemical control. I met a couple of other premeds, one was older, so we, we actually became good friends, did many things outside of school. But it was really good to study with somebody who worked very hard, who was focused, who was a little bit older. And that was really helpful for me at that level.

Q:
Did you ever use any school provided tutoring?

A:
My university offered a chemistry tutor. Forty hours a week there was a graduate student for the general chemistry courses who would answer questions. And I would seek their help. You would have to see who was doing the help and which graduate student it was. Some did not understand English very well. I would avoid them and go to the ones that I knew were good chemistry tutors. Other than that I did not use any resources.

Q:
You already touched on your advisement. It seems you had a quality advisor. How else did you use your advisor besides planning your course work?

A:
She was very helpful to me. I was very fortunate in my first biology course, my first semester back at Virginia Tech. She said to us in opening day of class, "Any of you going to professional school, I want you to come by my office and I want to get to know you. I

want to get to know what your goals are and I want you talk about them. Because I don't want you to come and ask me to write you a recommendation letter two years from now and all I know of you is a social security number and a grade."

So it is very important to get to know your basic science professors and let them get to know you especially those whose classes you're excelling in, because those are the people who you are going to ask to write recommendations for you and if those people don't know you, they can't write about you. So you have to give them an opportunity to get to know you.

Fortunately this woman told us up front to come and see her. I went to see her, got to know her very well and now she is a very good friend of mine. She advised me on course work. She advised me for professors to take courses from. She pointed me in the direction of different resources on and off campus. She also introduced me to another faculty member that I never took a course from, but who sat down and advised me concerning my goals. And both he and my primary premed advisor sat down with me with my AMCAS essay and gave me their perspective as basic science professors about what I was writing about.

She hooked me up with a general practitioner who invited me to see his practice. He took my wife and me out to dinner with his wife so she could get some feedback from the wife of a physician. He spent a lot of time with me.

Q:
Obviously you worked with this primary care doctor. What other medically related experiences did you participate in?

A:
That is a good question. When I was preparing myself as an applicant, I felt that I needed to either do lab research or get some practical experience. I am more interested in clinical medicine than research, therefore I chose the practical experience route. The opportunities weren't too great. The school had a preceptorship program but I could not be involved with it because I wasn't a full time undergraduate student. So I chose to become certified as an EMT in the State of Virginia. So I took a night course certification course.

Q:
At the same time you are doing MBA and your prereqs?

A:

That was the year before my wife joined me in Virginia. So I did not really have a life outside of school and work. But I took the course and was certified during my first semester of Virginia Tech. I was picked up by the local squad, not the university rescue squad which was student run, but the local town's rescue squad and I ran with them as an EMT as an ambulance driver for two years. I was able to get a lot of hands on experience. I chose the EMT route because, rather than being an orderly and being in a hospital and being told what to do and not being able to do too much, as an EMT you get a lot of hands on experience. You get a lot of responsibility for direct patient care and that was very challenging and very rewarding. I think it was a really good experience.

Q:

How about non medical activities?

A:

With my background I've done a lot. I had a lot of extracurricular activities that I could talk about prior going to Virginia Tech. Every base that I have been on I have played on the varsity volleyball team. So I have somewhat of a sports background. I have coached volleyball and basketball. At Virginia Tech I coached a basketball team. A midshipman basketball team. The Naval midshipman that we were training had a team and I coached that team. I played intramurals at Virginia Tech, played a little bit of basketball, played a lot of volleyball outside of that. Plus through the Navy , I had a lot of other kind of work experience, volunteer experience, volunteering at a day care center, to work with kids. Couple of things like that.

Q:

On to the MCAT. First of all, when do you think people should take it, and when did you take it?

A:

I took it in March prior to the summer I was going to apply. I recommend that people take it as soon as they have taken all the required courses. You have to have taken organic, you have to have taken chemistry and biology at the minimum. If you are going to take other courses that are going to build on those then you can wait a little bit longer to take the exam. But you need to take it in March. If you wait to take it in August and you are applying that year, you are way behind. And you'll hurt your chances at a lot of schools. You may still get in, but you are not going to have the opportunities you would have if you have gone and done it early. So I highly recommend that they take it in March of the year they are going to apply.

Q:
Did you take any review course?

A:
I took the Kaplan course. I chose that course because it was structured. I only had the basic bare minimum prerequisites. And I wanted somebody to tell me what to focus on. I hadn't had physics in eight years so I wanted to be able to take a review book, which they have, and take a course and have them point at the things that I needed to look at. I also was real happy with that program because they offered a lot of review material, a lot of practice tests, where you could kind of put yourself in a "testing situation" to really prepare yourself. The half length MCAT test that you take with them I think are very helpful. Because they almost put you in what I call a game situation. To help prepare you.

Q:
Besides Kaplan, how did you organize your study plan for the MCAT and how long did you study for?

A:
I took it in March, late March. I studied starting in January when I came back for that spring semester. The recommendation that I have is that this test is very important. Your performance on this test is very important. If you are taking semester courses and you finish the semester before Christmas, go to the Kaplan center. If you are going to take this course, pay for the books early so you can take them home with you over Christmas. No one wants to study over Christmas but if you are taking courses that spring, and I personally lightened up my load by one course that spring to allow some more time to study. If you're taking courses, if you're working, there is not a lot of time to prepare. So if you get those books and you have a couple of weeks where you are not in school, whether you're working or on vacation, spend time studying those books. Because the course comes real fast and there is no way to do everything that they recommend for in the nine to ten weeks that you have. So that I really recommend. I also recommend that you lighten up your schedule to prepare for it.

Q:
Anything else that you did to prepare for the MCAT?

A:
One thing that I did for the MCAT that was really helpful for me, is that I took a digital egg timer, one of those digital kitchen timers, I took it apart and deactivated the alarm so it wouldn't beep. But it had nice big digital numbers on it and you could set it up to count down. So if it was a forty-five minute exam, an hour exam, you could count down for you and that really helped me pace myself. I used it in the exam. And I used it to practice. The countdown with nice big digital numbers tells exactly what you have left. It really helped me to pace myself to make sure that I was getting every block of material done. So I finished the exam.

Q:
Now off to the AMCAS application . The non-essay part of the AMCAS I think is quite important, just like the essay part and it sounds like you had more than enough to fill up that small limited space. With all that you've done, how did you choose what to include and what to emphasize?

A:
What I tried to do with the AMCAS non-essay part was distinguish myself from a traditional medical student. I kind of looked at the AMCAS application as a way to market myself to a school. I had to show them what I did that was different than everyone else. The activities, the professional work experience, those sort of things. I listed and emphasized those things that would make more of impact. For example when I was flying in the Navy I was a mission commander, I was a combat crew mission commander. I felt that was important and it made me stand out. A lot of my military awards don't really make sense to a nonmilitary person so I didn't put a lot of my military awards, but I did put a lot of scholastic awards in the awards section. Extracurricular activities and those kind of things, I wanted to show both athletic participation and leadership and coaching to show that I wasn't just somebody that stuck his nose in a book but that I did take charge and show some leadership. So I tried to distinguish myself from the traditional student. You can guess that my work experience really focused on things that I had done in the Navy that were unique. So that's really ly how I tried to use that space.

Q:
When they asked you about your work experience in the navy you
tried to exemplify your leadership.

A:
Correct. One other little point about that section that I think is really important is to type it out on a copy of the AMCAS application
first. Be very detail specific and very exacting because that will
show a professional approach. If you have misspellings, mispunc-
tuation, the astute observer is going to pick up on that and anything
that makes you look bad is going to hurt you. So not only are you
very exacting but have everything proofread by somebody other
than yourself. A lot of times when you proofread your own work
you see what you thought you put down instead of what you really put down. Of course my wife was able to do all that for me.

Q:
What did you write about in your essay?

A:
In the essay, I kind of wanted to distinguish myself. I felt that it was
necessary to explain my career change, especially since I was an
older student. The people that are reviewing you might say well
this person just decided that they want to go into medicine and is
going to change his mind in five or ten years. A university doesn't
want to invest in you and train you as physician unless you are
going to go out and make a good name for them, because there are
plenty of other candidates who are going to that. So I felt that I
needed my career change. I felt that I needed to justify my MBA,
my pursuit of an MBA. I felt that I needed to once again bring out
some of the things that I had done in the Navy. I talked about some
of the unique experiences that I have had that other people have
not experienced.

And I brought out some of the life experiences that I have
had that I think make me a stronger, better person and a better candidate for medical school than probably some other people. Like
being in charge, being a combat air crew commander, being a division officer in the Navy. I had a forty-four man division that I was
in charge of, responsible for not only seeing that they did their
work, but in the Navy you are responsible for the performance,
training and welfare of your personnel. So that meant that when
one of my guys was in jail, it was me who went to bail them out.
When one of my guys was in trouble, it was me who had to talk
them about that, council them about being separated, and their

responsibilities as a father and husband even though they weren't living with the person, but to financially support the person... those sort of things that your average manager in a corporation does not have to worry about. So I kind of stressed those things.

Also, I had a couple of things happen. Our squadron lost two airplanes in a midair collision. I lost some good friends and lost some people who worked for me. I lost my boss on those air-planes. That sort of life experience, for me personally made me a stronger person. I kind of discussed those sort of things. I also addressed the fact that I was personally interested in clinical med-icine and that I wanted, and I still am primarily interested in pri-mary practice. I knew that hurt me at some schools that I applied to but I felt it was important to be honest about those things.

Q:
Obviously you probably had a number of secondary applications to fill out. Give me your general impressions of those applications.

A:
I used the shotgun approach when I decided to apply to medical school. I kind of planned and thought it out and took a very orga-nized approach to apply once. I was going to apply one year and that's it. I was at a point in my life this was my goal, this was my career change, but I had a fall back plan. If it didn't work out I was-n't going to spin my wheels a couple of years if it didn't work out. I set myself up to be the best candidate that I could then I went for it once and that was it. With that spirit on my primary AMCAS application I applied to 20 schools, listed 20 schools. Of those 20 I received 18 supplemental. Of those eighteen I returned twelve.

So it is really hard for me to really focus in on what ques-tions that were asked. But I think a common theme that would come up for me personally, once again I dwelled upon my experi-ence that made me different.

I didn't dwell on my experience as an EMT. I just stated the fact that I did this to gain direct patient contact, direct patient care responsibility and that I had done it for so long. Because there are a lot of EMTs out there who are applying to medical school. I dwelt on the things that made me different. When they asked me a question I thought about how I could weave this in to my professional experience, my navy background. A lot of the questions from a lot schools although they weren't the same had the same sort of content and I just cut and pasted a lot of things. I would take a thought from my AMCAS essay and expand it. I would take an answer from another question on another supplemental and change it and make it appropriate for the question that was asked. It saved a lot of time, it saved a lot of effort.

With the computer it was real nice. I worked on the supplemental using the computer instead of hand typing them and that worked out really well. I would make copies of the secondary applications. I would run the copy through my printer, make sure I had everything properly lined up and aligned and then I had a backup if I screwed up the one they wanted me to send back to them. Once I had a good product I ran the original through. I printed directly on the application and that worked out really well.

For the AMCAS hard card, I typed everything but the essay. I took the essay to Kinko's and they were able to run the hard card through their printers, actually print the essay on the card. Made sure I had a couple extras.

Q:
Did you update your applications at all after you sent in the secondaries?

A:
It wasn't really necessary for me to do that because I sent in the AMCAS right away the first day they would accept them. I think they would accept them on the June 15th. I overnighted mine the 14th. And if you will recall from that year if that's what you did, the MCAT scores weren't back yet. But I felt that it was important to get there. It gets in line, it's got to get in line. Everyday that you're behind somebody else it lowers your chances. I overnighted it on the 14th so it arrived on the 15th. Then my supplemental were coming back all summer.

So all my summer courses were MBA courses. It didn't change my GPA, my MBA GPA would remain the same. I was done with my prereqs. I had already scheduled the histology course for the fall. I didn't even know about the neurochemical course that I would take in the spring of that year. So I didn't feel it was necessary to update with a couple of grades during the summer time in courses that didn't matter. Courses that were already listed as intended courses.

One thing I did feel was important was for me to make kind of a clean break between what I did as an undergrad and my GPA which was good as an undergrad and what I did as a graduate student and in my post-bacc courses. I tried to make a clear difference, that I was a good student then, but I am an excellent student now. That would have been one reason to include more courses had I improved my GPA, but I did not improve it, it was a 4.0 so I could only hurt myself. So, I didn't feel it necessary to update.

Now there was one school, Loyola in Chicago, that wanted every semester updated grades. I think Emory wanted something like that too. And I satisfied those requirements. But I really didn't have anything new to add. All of my outstanding background non medical things were in the past. My grades didn't change. My medical experience didn't change. The only thing I might have added was I did some research as an MBA student and had a paper published. I might have updated that on application or two. That might have made a difference at the big research schools.

Q:
We discussed when to apply and that you think timing is important.

A:
Critical, not just important... critical.

Q:
How did you choose the schools that you applied to?

A:
I had a plan. In the spring before I applied I took the AMCAS publication and started reading about schools. And I used the stratified approach. I broke the schools down into the top ten schools, the next most competitive group and the other group, all the rest. And I made sure that when I selected those twenty schools, that I wanted to select a few of the top ten, a number of the most competitive, and I wanted to select a bunch of all the rest. So I was going for some long shots with the top ten and I was going for some pretty good possibilities with the middle group. With the lower group I had some essentially sure things especially the state schools. I am a resident of Florida so I applied to all four Florida state schools.

That spring I also wrote a form letter, easy to do on the computer, printed out form labels and everything for every one of those schools that I was going to apply on AMCAS and I requested a catalog. I think that is very important because when you read a school's catalog you kind of get an understanding for the philosophy of the school. And if you understand the philosophy of the school it is going to help you get an interview and it going to help you write a secondary application. It is going to help you answer questions and market yourself as the sort of student they are looking for.

Q:
Let's talk a little about recommendations. How did you choose the people that you elected to write your recommendations?

A:
The way that they did things at Virginia Tech, there was a premed advisory committee, which was a committee of about 20 professors, who would get together in the spring in panels of three and interview student prospectives. So they would interview you and mock interview you which gave you good practice and it enabled them to evaluate you on more than just your grades. In order to be in that program you had to have a minimum of three recommendation letters. After you went through that program one person who was on your committee of three would write your committee medical school recommendation letter for you.

I selected professors that I did well in their course, and professors who I knew personally, who knew me and who I felt respected me as a student and then asked them point blank, can you write me a good recommendation? Not will you write me a recommendation, not are you capable or not do you think I deserve a good recommendation, but can you write me a good recommendation. It's kind of a loaded question. I knew that I was a good student and I knew that they respected me or I thought that they did, but I also wanted to know if they were a good writer.

And I also focused on people that were going to be on that committee. People who had seen a lot of medical students and a lot of premeds. So those are the kind of people I had write the committee. Fortunately for me, my committee of three consisted of a professor that I worked with professionally as an instructor. We used to sit on academic review boards together as co-members of the board so that professor had seen me professionally. Another professor whose course that I had taken was someone I talked to outside the course and knew very well and I also ran on the EMT rescue squad with his daughter. So his daughter knew me from a paramedical professional light. And the other professor I had never met before. But that of those three the one professor whose course I had taken wrote the group letter for me and that is the letter that went to all the schools. So after you have gone through that process all I did was just give a medical school address to the secretary and the letter went out.

Q:
Did you have additional letters from different sources?

A:

Depending on the school. Some schools required additional letters. Some schools didn't. I went to my commanding officer.
Somebody I had worked with for three years who knew me very
well as an officer on a professional level, and knew of my academic background as a student. Someone who could shed a little
light on my professional performance. Who could say, I worked
with this guy and I have worked with a lot of guys like him and this
is where he falls out. I felt that was important at a lot of schools
and I sent that letter to a lot of schools. Schools like Stanford
require a letter from an MD, so there was an MD that I befriended
who was in the MBA course who was very helpful to me.

      He helped me review my AMCAS application also.   I
highly recommend that an MD review your AMCAS application
not just an academic type. Because your application is going to be
looked at by academics and MDs and they both look at the world
differently. So the academics gave me good advice, the MD gave
me good advice and help put things together. The MD was real
helpful as a last check because that MD can tell you if that letter
looks professional, whether it looks arrogant. Maybe you should-
n't say something in that way because although you mean it per-
fectly honestly it might look offensive to an MD. Always have that
AMCAS read by an MD.

      But he was also helpful in prepping me for interviews. He
asked me the tough ethical questions. Sat down and worked
through those with me. So he was very helpful. So those were the
kind of people. And he also wrote me a recommendation letter to
a couple of schools. And I asked the people that wrote recommendations for me to let me read their letters of recommendation.
I never saw the committee letter my school wrote. And I don't
know to this day what they wrote. The other letters I asked per-
mission to have a copy of because I want to know what they are
writing on me. It becomes helpful when you go for an interview if
you know what they have on you. You know exactly what you
wrote on the AMCAS, but you should also know what is written in
recommendation letters so you can either support them, or be prepared to answer a question that might come up from one of those
letters.

Q:

What were your different interviews like?

A:

Emory had a committee. Two MDs and one medical student interviewing three prospectives at once. That is the only committee interview that I had. Every other interview that I had at every other school was one on one. One thing I think that is really important if you're on a panel interview is to make sure you're attentive to the other students because while they are asking the other students questions they are going to watch you, and see whether or not you're rolling your eyes, yawning, how polite you're being to them. Because that, I think, is a peephole inside you as a person, your character.

Q:
Did you prepare for your interviews?

A:
As far as preparing for the interview I think dress is very important, you want to come off professionally. Fortunately as an MBA student, I was trained to present myself as a business type so I knew the right clothes to wear, I knew the right shoes and socks. What kind of suit to wear. You want to dress conservatively, professionally. You want to have a conservative image including professional hygiene, haircut, nail trim. If you just worked on the car over the weekend, make sure that all the grease is out from under your fingernails. The conservative professional is the key. You don't want to make a statement with your attire. That is not usually going to work in your favor.

As far as prepping for the interviews I think that is very important. You need to know the key issues, the important issues at the different schools. If the school is in a budget fight. If the school is downsizing. It is important to know these things. You're not going to get that kind of information from the school catalog. The catalog is going to tell you about the school goals and direction. For each school you need to know that going into the interview. They are going to ask you if you have any questions at the end of the interview in most cases. It is good to have a intelligent question about the school. Specific to the individual school, how does the school do this or how is the school addressing this issue.

You also need to know exactly what they have on you. So as many times as I read it, I always reread my AMCAS the night before or the morning before an interview. I always reread the secondary application the night before or the morning before. And I would practice questions. I practiced with classmates. I practiced with the MD I told you about. I practiced with myself. I am going to get a question on my navy past. I am going to get a question on why medicine. Why the MBA. I practiced those. So when they said why do you want to study medicine or the very tough questions, tell me your best trait and your worst trait. Or tell me three adjectives that describe you. You have to practice all those things out. Not that it comes out like you're reading from note cards but that it comes out that you thought it out so you have your thoughts together.

Q;
Anything else about interviews?

A:
Another thing I did is what I call preflight. Another navy flying term. Preflight everything. Before I left town for an interview I made sure that I had my interview outfit. What you can call built to man. I laid it out all on the bed. Suit, shirt, ties, socks, underwear, shoes. Everything I need. Raincoat if necessary. Overcoat if it is winter time. Umbrella. Lay everything out. Also for me I have some allergies occasionally. I made sure that I had my allergy medicine. And I took it prophylactically that morning. Because the last thing that I want to do was sneeze on an interviewer or all through an interview. So I built a man, packed a man. If I was flying I got to the airport early. Took a good book. What I typically would do, is get to the interview site the night before, and I would scout out the interview site. I would know exactly where I was going to park the next morning. Exactly where the building was the next morning, exactly where the admissions office was. So I didn't leave anything to chance. So I wasn't going to be late, because if you're late you're setting a bad first impression.

At every school I was seriously interested in, I really talked to the students. I spent time talking to the students. I talked to the professors. When I would go for an interview there were two things going on- I was interviewing them and they were interviewing me. So I asked a lot of questions of professors. I talked to faculty members. I talked to students. I got students names and numbers so that I could call them back. And I very discriminately looked at the facilities to see if this was where I wanted to go to school for the next four years. Here at Northwestern when I came for my interview I went on a tour. And they toured all the academic facilities but we didn't tour the hospital. So I sat down with Dean Brown, the dean of Admissions and said "Dean Brown, I want to see the hospital." And she found Dean Berry to take me to see the hospital. So I got a tour from Dean Barry to see the hospital.

I think it is really important to ask the questions, be prepared with a list of questions. If there is something you are not sure of ask. If there is point in the way the curriculum is taught ask. It shows that number one you care and that you looked it up. That you're interested. You need to feel them out. I thought about it every site. Do I want to live around here? Do I want to commute to here? Is this going to be a comfortable for my wife and me? Is she going to be able to find work? So I thought about all these things when I went to the interviews.

Q:
How did you choose where to accept?

A:
A long story. I had twelve supplementals, I was invited for interviews at all but one of those schools. I went to six interviews of those 11 invitations. I was accepted at 4 of those places, wait listed at two of those places, and one of them I withdrew from. The other one I stayed on the wait list until it was pretty much between here and there. And that school was Duke. A big part of the reason why I am in the Chicago area is that my family is around here and I have been away from them for eight years, seeing them once or twice a year. And this was an opportunity for my wife and me to live near them. Her family is in California. There was another very similar program at Pittsburgh where I was accepted. Very similar to Northwestern in many ways. And those two were pretty close. I was also accepted at the University of Chicago and was all ready to go there. I was all ready to go there. I was accepted at Loyola, but was not interested in Loyola after being at the University of Chicago.

I am here because of a lot of reasons. The curriculum is a big part of the reason why I am here. The clinical focus is a little better here than it is down at University of Chicago. I'm not interested in academic medicine, if I was I would be there. They recruited me very aggressively down there. The facilities are gorgeous. They opened their building three years ago. So brand new laboratories, brand-new classrooms. The anatomy lab does not smell bad. Beautiful, beautiful facilities. Great faculty, great basic science faculty. A lot of research opportunities, I was almost there. But it was the students that I talked to that brought me here.

Q:
What was special about the students at Northwestern?

A:

The students at U of C were very impressive and very enthusiastic. But the students here I felt were happier. And that's for me, being married, having had a life after school before coming to medical school, I wanted a school where I knew I was going to be happy student and not be beat up with eight hours of classroom a day. Which is essentially what they do down there with the labs.

Q:

Is there anything else you want to add?

A:

Timing is critical, planning is critical. If you're a nontraditional student you probably don't have a lot of time to mess around and to apply for a few years in a row so you must make sure you're going to do everything that you can to make yourself a good candidate. And the only other recommendation I would have is be aggressive and ask the questions at any medical school that you are interested in - ask what do I need to do to make me a better candidate. If you're dead set on going to a school get an interview with the Dean of Admissions at that school, well before you go into the process and find out what they look for in a student so you can set yourself up and then market yourself.

One other recommendation that comes along with professionalism is that it is proper, appropriate, and professional to send a handwritten thank you to an interviewer after the interviewer has seen you. Etiquette would require that it be sent the day after the interview. If not hand delivered, then put in the mail the day after the interview. So what you should probably do is to get a bunch of thank you cards maybe with your school seal on them, if you have a unique school seal, being from Virginia Tech which does not put out a lot of premeds that was kind of unique. Handwritten thank you, proper spelling of the name of the person, proper address, get the address before you leave the admissions office. Talk to the receptionist and ask for an address for the people who interviewed you. If you have to you can always send them care of the admissions office. Handwrite it. Sign it and make sure your signature is legible so they know who is sending them a thank you. And try to put something personal in every one. If you are interviewed by a committee, by two or three Drs. don't send a form, because they are going to get together and say "hey I got a thank you from Bill McCullough. Oh, so did I. What did yours say? Well that is what mine said." Try to personalize them, to show that you picked up on some personal interaction.

146

It is a sign of professionalism, it stands out to me because having interviewed medical students for school, I noticed who sent thank yous and who didn't. And the Thank you whether you like it or not, make you feel good, make you think that they appreciated the time you put into this. Because all the committee members are volunteers, not one of them is paid except maybe the Dean of Admissions to interview people. Write them a thank you. It is going to make them feel better and it is going to make each of them remember you.

Q:
Great points. Thanks a lot Bill.

Interview Twelve - - Heidi Memmel

HEIDI MEMMEL: Heidi is twenty seven years old. She graduated from Northwestern University with a degree in German Studies. Before medical school she worked for an executive recruiting firm as research manager and executive recruiter in the petroleum industry.

Q:
What did you do before you came to medical school?

A:
I worked for about four and half years at an executive recruiting firm. I started out as a research assistant, then became a research manager, then worked as a recruiter for the retail petroleum industry. When I decided I wanted to come back to medical school, the time commitment was a little bit too much as a recruiter so I offered to stay on as a research assistant if they would be flexible with my hours. They offered me a job back as the research manager.

Q:
So how did you make your decision to go back to medical school?

A:
I think it was something I had been thinking about for years. I started out in undergrad as a premed. I dropped the premed courses early in my sophomore year. Then by the time I graduated I was kind of kicking myself that I didn't finish, just to give myself that option to go to medical school.

Q:
So you made your decision while you were working?

A:
I think so. I had been thinking about it since graduation. But I probably made my decision two years out of school. Probably 1992. I started classes, post-baccalaureate classes in late '92, about 6 months after I made the decision to go back.

Q:
What type of premed program did you enroll in?

A:

I was enrolled in Loyola's post-bacc premed program. I started out taking chemistry the first year. I took biology over the first summer and then organic chemistry and physics the second year. I took the MCATs at the end of the second year.

Q:

Did you have a way you chose your classes other than your work schedule?

A:

They had classes that were set up for people that were working during the days. I pretty much just followed that format. I knew that I wanted to take chemistry first because that was the most basic science. Then take biology over a compacted 12 week summer course. With that course I had a midterm every other Friday.

Q:

How many courses did you take at once?

A:

The most I took was two, plus labs, plus 5 days of work a week, plus studying for the MCATS on the weekends.

Q:

As far as the materials you used to study for your premed classes, which were the most valuable to you?

A:

I studied from my notes. Everyone borrowed my notes. I had old exams and my class exams to study for the finals. Also old exams from previous years. They were always floating around in class. For one of the professors they were extremely helpful. One of the professors I had also supplied old exams. As I think about it, the other one didn't because he used same questions over again.

Q:

Did you use study groups?

A:

Not really. I studied on my own because pretty much everyone in my class worked during the days so it was kind of hard to coordinate study groups.

Q:
Did you use the school advisor at all?

A:
I did, but I did not find it too helpful. The school advisor interviews you before you start classes. Then he tells you that you shouldn't go. He gives you the reasons why. He totally discourages you and then at the end he interviews you again and he writes a letter of recommendation for you. First of all, his questions are: "If you were a tree, what kind of tree would you be and why?" "If you were an element on the periodic chart, what element would you be and why? " Instead of compiling all your answers to his questions in a concise well thought out recommendation, he lists your answers. So I did not find him too helpful.

Q:
Did you use the school advisement center for medical school applications?

A:
Yes, I did use it for that and it was helpful to have a central place to coordinate all of the recommendations and information.

Q:
I know you worked full time, but what extracurricular activities did you do that were medically related?

A:
I volunteered in an emergency department for four years. Once a week.   Other things I did were work at burn camp for a couple of years. I was also on the junior board of Big Brothers/Big Sisters for Metropolitan Chicago. And I also did other things like Special Olympics.

Q:
So you did have a significant amount of extracurricular activities. Did you think your experiences helped your application?

A:
I think so, because it gave me additional experiences and things to write about. Application essays. AMCAS essays, personal statements etc.

Q:
The MCAT. When do you think you should take it?

A:
Spring. Definitely spring. Every year in Illinois, there is a big convention of all the medical school admissions directors and admissions boards. Or not necessarily the admissions board but a representative from the admissions department of each medical
school. It is a day or two day event. It was actually really useful.
One presenter spoke on how to write your personal statement.
There are little seminars for whatever you are interested in. If you
are interested in financial aid or writing an effective personal statement, or studying for the MCAT. And admissions directors talk on
different subjects . I asked them the question about my situation.
I work five days a week and take classes five nights a week. I am
wondering if I should run the risk of not having enough time to
study for the MCAT, taking it in the spring. Or putting it off for the
fall. They said definitely take it in the spring. If you can squeeze
in the time , take it in the spring and get your application in that
much earlier.

Q:
Did you take any review courses?

A:
No.

Q:
So how did you organize your studying?

A:
I did have some of the materials from Kaplan. All the books. Some
of them were useful. I kind of picked and chose between topics.
Also, I used the Flowers guide for some of the topics. Detailed, but
really good. On subjects that I needed more work, I went back to
old notes and college textbooks. For some of the other ones I used
Kaplan. For verbal I used Kaplan. Also I did a lot of the MCAT old
tests.

Q:
How long did you study for?

A:
I just studied on the weekends. I think I tried to study maybe six or

eight hours a day on the weekend. Probably for a couple of
months.

Q:
For the AMCAS application what did you try to emphasize or
include in the non essay part? Did you try to present a certain
image?

A:
Not really. I think my background and activities presented me as
pretty well rounded. I was a German studies major with an eco-
nomics minor. I really had nothing to with medicine before I started volunteering.

Q:
For your essay, what did you write about and how did you organize
it?

A:
Some of the advice that we received from an admissions director at
that convention, was that admissions committees are relatively
conservative. Try to stick along those lines. Try to let them see who
you are as a person. Not just "This is why I want to go to medical
school, because I am a wonderful person, I love working with people, blah, blah, blah." This is what 90% of medical students write
about. They want to see more of the picture of yourself. Of your
past experiences, what your reactions to the experiences were and
how it affected you. So I wrote about an experience at the trauma
center that I was working at. Just about how a man came into the
hospital just after his wife had been in a car accident. I think he
was in his nineties. And I just sat in the waiting room for half an
hour while he waited for his family. I think it ended up being a
pretty good essay. A couple of admissions people where I interviewed commented that they liked it.

Q:
So you tried to pick one event instead of trying to tell everything
that is on your resume. You tried to show a little of your personal
side?

A:
Right. I tried to pick an experience rather than just repeat what I
had already said on the non-essay portion.

Q:

Can you remember your general impression of your secondary applications?

A:

I tried to use them the same way as the AMCAS essay or personal statement. I tried not to repeat things that were on the AMCAS. I tried not to repeat lists of activities or lists of stuff. I tried to more relate it to a personal aspect rather than just background and history.

Q:

Did you update your application after your secondary or did you send extra stuff?

A:

I did. The only additional things I had to send were updated grades from the Physics lab that I took after the MCAT. That was all that I updated.

Q:

And so by taking the MCAT early you were able to apply early.

A:

I think that was a huge help, and one of the doctors commented that it was great that I am interviewing early, because later on spots are so limited it is hard to pick and choose between people who are all qualified and who are all great applicants.

Q:

As far as the schools that you chose to apply to, how did you choose?

A:

Well, I wanted to stay here in Chicago and I am still officially a resident of Wisconsin because Wisconsin has this goofy rule that if you graduate from high school in Wisconsin, spent over so many years in Wisconsin, and your parents still live in Wisconsin then they will consider you as a resident. So I applied to the two Wisconsin schools. I applied to everything in Chicago and then Georgetown and Case-Western. I chose Case Western on the recommmendation of my Loyola advisor. They look kindly at post-bacc applicants.

Q:
How many schools did you apply to?

A:
Ten or eleven.

Q:
How did you choose the people that you got your recommendations from?

A:
Our office, I don't know if this is similar for most medical students or at most undergraduate schools advising their students on applying to medical school. But they only wanted us to submit a certain number- no more than 5 recommendations. Two from science professors, one from another professor, and one from a supervisor. So I had one from my direct supervisor from the company I was working for. I had two from my post-bacc professors whose courses I had just taken. And one from Northwestern undergrad from one of my professors in my major who I had taken 4 classes with. Oh and then one from my volunteer positions.

Q:
So you did get one from the hospital you volunteered at? Who did you get to write it?

A:
I initially asked someone from the volunteer department, but all they sent was a letter that said this is Heidi Memmel who had been a volunteer for four years. So I got one of the attending physicians to write me one.

Q:
Now as far as your interviews went, do you remember the different types?

A:
I do. At Loyola, they had us interview with two physicians. I had an interview with an Ob/Gyn. and a neonatalogist. The interview with the neonatologist was a half open-half closed file interview. They don't see your grades and they don't see your scores. All they see is your list of activities, where you are from, and your personal statement. That interview went really well. The interview before that with the OB/Gyn I think that went all right too. It was not quite

as comfortable, but it went all right.

My interviews at Rush, one went terrible. We were in this tiny room. I think it was a closed file interview. I had a really hard time understanding this man because his English was not very good. He was asking me questions like "if I were the President of the United States how would I change the Health care system?" I told him my answer, explained it. And then he said "but what else?" So I thought of a couple more things. He kept asking me what else. Then after going on to another question, and then five minutes later, then he says "how I wanted you to answer or how you should have answered was this". I thought "okay, this was my interview, how I would do things." So that did not go very well.

Q:
Were there any questions that stuck out in your mind that they asked that you thought were really good?

A:
One question was in a panel interview : If you had to ask someone an interview question in this row, what would you ask? And from then on, everybody thought they meant hypothetical situation. So the next seven questions were all stupid hypothetical situation that got more and more detailed and more and more ridiculous.

Q:
How did you dress?

A:
I wore a suit.

Q:
How did you prepare for your interviews?

A:
I have a packet of interview questions. I went through a lot of those.

Q:
Where did you get those?

A:
From other people who applied to medical school as well as the premed office at Loyola. The premed office at Loyola had com-

ments from medical students that had interviewed at different schools in the past. For example, for Northwestern, they had a packet of forms filled out from medical students who had interviewed there which included questions like "What types of questions you were you asked, was the interview comfortable, etc." Just so you know what to expect when going in, which is kind of nice. I also tried to prepare by reading or keeping abreast of the health care status and health care policy reform. That was a hot topic. I also prepared by knowing my background well. By knowing dates of when I did things. For example- I was on the sailing team from 89-90 and just stuff like that. I also prepared by trying to learn more about each school. You know, what their curriculum is, what really stands out.

Q:
Do you have any general recommendations for people who are applying to medical school?

A:
General recommendations: apply early, have someone read over your essays, spellcheck them. And the biggest thing I think is to apply early. If you can't change anything and are already past the point of adding other activities, get your application in early and apply to a lot of schools.

I do have one recommendation about the waiting list. If you are on the waiting list keep contacting the school, send more information, send grades, send another letter of recommendation, submit a letter of why you really want to go to that school, call every other week. The schools that I have talked to look highly upon remaining in contact because it shows them interest. They would rather admit someone from the waiting list who they know really is going to go there and not back out at the last minute when they get called from the waiting list from another school.

Q:
How did you choose Northwestern?

A:
Well, it is in Chicago. It is the school I really wanted to go to because of its academic reputation, it is both primary care and specialty oriented and it is very prominent in both. I wanted to go somewhere that gave me options. If you go to some place like Rush, primary care is such a big deal there and I wanted to have at least have the option to chose my specialty. I did not want to be

already programmed to be on a certain path by going to a certain school.

Q:
Thanks Heidi.

Interview Thirteen — Elizabeth Weil

ELISABETH WEIL: Elizabeth is forty years old. She graduated from Colorado College in 1978. After working for a number of years, she went back to graduate school at Northwestern and received a master's degree in Speech Pathology in 1984. After graduating, she practiced as a speech pathologist for two years in Florida and then at the Rehabilitation Institute of Chicago.

A:
My name is Elizabeth R. Weil, and I just turned 40.

Q:
Can you talk a little bit about what you did before you made the transition to medical school?

A:
I was working as a speech language pathologist. I graduated from college in '78, took a few years off and kind of bummed around, did odd jobs. I went back to graduate school, actually went to Northwestern, got a master's degree in speech pathology. So I had been working since 1984 doing speech pathology mostly with neurological patients, people with strokes and brain injuries. I worked for 2 years for a private practice in Florida and the rest of the time here at RIC.

Q:
So what made you make the decision to go back to medical school?

A:
I loved my job, I loved the people I worked with. I worked on a small team. There were 9 people on my team who worked on a day program for people with head injuries. I really liked my job, but when I thought about doing it every day for the rest of my life, I just couldn't see doing that. I liked my job a lot so I didn't want to just find a new job in speech pathology because I thought I probably wouldn't enjoy it as much as the one I already had.

     I think I've always been the kind of person who changed what I was doing every few years. That's what I'm doing now. My job just wasn't challenging for me anymore. And I didn't find it stimulating enough to create challenges for myself in my job like by doing teaching courses, I did a little of that, or doing research.

None of that interested me really. So I decided very suddenly, actually, to go to medical school.

Q:
And what steps did you take toward that goal?

A:
I didn't do a good job of researching it. I mean I knew I needed to take courses just to take the MCAT. It was about the middle of summer when I decided that I wanted to start taking some premed courses. My idea always was, Okay, I'll take some courses and see how that goes. If I don't like it, I'll just go back to my job. I found out that Loyola has a post-baccalaureate premed program. I called the man who was in charge and went up there and talked to him. He got me into school right away. Like this was in the middle of summer — the deadline, if there was a deadline, was coming up very soon but it wasn't too late. So I got into school in the fall.

Q:
So you went through a post-bacc program at Loyola?

A:
Yeah. What I did was take a leave of absence from my job at RIC because I didn't know if I'd want to go back, if I would quit school and go back to work. I didn't want to lose the benefits. By taking a leave of absence, you can still build vacation and all that. So I wasn't working at all. I started by taking 3 classes - biology, physics and general chemistry. And I sort of freaked out after about - I can't remember, it was whenever the deadline is to drop a class. I decided I would drop one.   I had decided to drop physics because I just couldn't - I didn't think I could take all 3 of those classes at once. My plan was to take all 3 of them and then to take organic chemistry over the summer and apply within that time frame. And I changed my mind and decided to take 2 classes, not to take anything during the summer, and then to take 2 more classes which is what I ended up doing.

Q:
Is that the advice you'd give to somebody?

A:
I think it just depends on the individual. It delayed me a year, but in the long run, what's a year? I'm already one of the oldest people in the class. Another year's not going to change that. And I got

in, I did really well.

People tried to convince me not to drop the class. Other people in the classes said oh, you can do it, you can take three. And they're probably right. I probably could have, but I don't know if I would have done as well. I know it wouldn't have been as enjoyable a year . And I know that taking things over the summer is really hard. I don't know if I would recommend that unless you're in a real big hurry because I know that people say that you don't learn - all you're doing is cramming things into your head. You don't hang on to them. So I don't know if I recommend taking anything over the summer. It's too short.

Q:
As far as your classes go, did you have any specific methodology in choosing the teachers?

A:
Not the first year. I didn't know any of them. I did it more by the times. I'm a morning person so I went to lectures in the morning. I actually had pretty good luck. I changed both of them for the second semester, actually because I had to, neither of them were continuing to teach the second semester. So actually that might be one thing to do, to find someone who's going to be teaching all year. Make sure you like them. If you don't think you'll like them, it's OK to change professors after the first semester. If you change, you have to get adjusted to a whole new teaching style in the middle of the year. Some people might like that, some people might not. You have to start all over figuring out what the tests are going to be like. Sometimes I think I worked harder at Loyola in that program than I did the first year of medical school because you had to get A's. And I was so overwhelmed by everything I had to know to take the MCAT.

Q:
It's a lot of information.

A:
Right. It is a lot of information.

Q:
What did you use to study for your coursework? Did you use the textbooks, old tests, notes? What did you find helpful?

A:

I actually did all of the reading or at least most of it, a lot more than I could do the first year of medical school. There was just more time because I was just taking two classes. So I really did do all of the reading and I studied from my notes and some from the book and some from these really nice summaries my organic chemistry professor would put together.

I also went to tutoring which I thought was really helpful. I was getting A's and I was still going to tutoring. The classes were big and I went to a really small liberal arts college and a small graduate school program, and it was the first time I ever had classes with over 30 people in them. And I'm not very good about going after hours to office hours and asking professors questions because I usually went home. I didn't study at school. I thought it was sort of a pain, so I always had questions. So I decided to take advantage of the tutoring program — it was offered by the school, it was a free tutoring program. I know I had a guy for my physics tutor who was just great. He was also in the premed program, post-bacc premed, and he was actually in chemistry class and was my physics tutor — that was kind of fun. It just helped me to have somebody to ask questions who I knew knew the answer, as opposed to just asking somebody in my class.

Q:
Did you use study groups?

A:

I pretty much studied on my own. I didn't go to any study groups or anything like that. That's just the way I study better, alone I guess.

Q:
Tell me about the advisement you received for both your applications and planning a class schedule.

A:

At Loyola, there was a man who doesn't work there anymore, but who was the head of the program, this post-baccalaureate program. He helped me with the scheduling. I think he actually did encourage me to do two course, one year and two courses the other year. So originally, I wasn't going by his advice. I was going to take 3 classes and then one over the summer because I was in a hurry, but it didn't work.

They had programs at Loyola, lecture series and things for

the students in the program. On medical ethics and things like that.
I actually went to some of those, partially out of interest, partially
so that my advisor would see me there because he wrote a cover
letter for the letters of recommendation from the faculty at Loyola.
I had heard that you had to get on his good side so he'll write you
a good letter or at least so he knows who you are because it's a really huge program. So I went to some of those things.

Then towards the end, we actually had an interview with
him so that he could write you a cover letter. We had this mini
interview and he asked questions. Some of it was sort of practice
for interviewing and getting into medical school. The questions
were pretty ridiculous that he asked, but I guess it helped him write
the letter.

Additionally, they did have some panels of people who
had gotten into school and came back and talked about what they
had written on their applications. I think I went to those things
the first year I was there and the second year when I should have
been going, I was too busy so I didn't go to any of them. Actually
now that I think of it, they did have a lot of meetings like that where
they talked about applications, what you should write and what
you shouldn't write and how to do the essays. Actually, that was a
really helpful part of going to a school that had an actual program.

Q:
Did your program have a central recommendation file?

A:
Yeah they had a file for letters of recommendation. So that was all
on file. Then you'd ask them to send your file out.

Q:
Tell me a little bit about your extra-curricular activities. Did you do
anything else? I know that you were involved in medicine on a
daily basis.

A:
No, you see, for that kind of thing, I really didn't emphasize much
on my application. I figured that was either for people who were
just out of college so they hadn't worked at all or who had done
some spectacular thing in addition to whatever job they had had. I
basically had my job. I was pretty active for a while in a local theater that is run by people who are now my friends. I think I mentioned that a little bit, but I hadn't really done anything that I
thought would get me in. And I hadn't done a lot of extra-curric-

ular activities in college or in high school. I mean I had done some, but nothing outstanding. And I think I mentioned I put down the little things I had done where there was room, but I didn't worry too much about that. I think people had said that was really more for people just out of school who hadn't had a chance to work or do anything else.

Q:
Let's talk about the MCAT a little bit. First of all, when did you take it and when do you recommend that people take it?

A:
I took it in April. I highly recommend taking it in the spring just because your chances of getting interviews are much better. That's just the timetable most people go by. If you apply in fall, you'll be interviewing later in the year I think and they'll have accepted people already. You'll be like squeaking in if you're lucky. I think you have to do better, score better, to get in if you take it in the fall.

Q:
I would agree with you completely. Did you take any review courses?

A:
I took the Kaplan course because I was having a hard time making myself study. It was a lot of money, but I really thought I needed the structure of going someplace and having some structure to push me to help me study. The review materials, they give you these books, one for each subject, those were good. Those were fine. I actually used those. And review questions or test questions that I think you can get with that, I used all those. But they also have all these practice tests you can take and then you go listen to these tapes where they go over and explain the answers. I found those took more time than they were worth to me. They went into too much detail. And that's sort of a big part of what you're paying for I think. So I didn't even do much of that. I did more of going to the actual class, the review class which was once a week, I did it for 2-3 hours every Saturday morning listening to this really weird guy go over all these facts we had to know. But I found that real helpful. I don't know if it changed my scores at all.

Q:
How long did you study for?

A:
Probably 2 months. I wasn't working at all.   I wasn't on any big schedule. I was just trying to go over things. Mostly I think I used the review materials in the books. I did do a lot of practice tests.

            Also I did the old MCAT tests which were available.   I thought those were really helpful. I thought those were really good. I did all the practice tests. I thought that was a good way to study. And I spent a lot of time timing myself which is something that they recommended at Kaplan, trying to do test questions as fast as you would have to do them for the test. Like I would take a set number of questions and figure out how much time I would have if I was taking the test and I gave myself a time limit. I thought that was really important because then you know how fast you need to go when you're taking it. That's really the hardest part .

Q:
What did you list on the non-essay part of the AMCAS application?

A:
Well I did get this award from the Communicative Disorders Department at Northwestern, the graduate school had the honor of the department which is for being the top student for 2 years. And I definitely put that down.   I did put down the theater and just things I like to do.

Q:
What did you do in the theater?

A:
I had been the box office manager.   I didn't do any acting, I just sat in on rehearsals. All of the plays that they did there, people wrote themselves and then produced. So I kind of gave advice about how things were going, what I liked and didn't like. I some- times I did tech stuff like ran the lights and props.

Q:
Do you remember what you wrote in your essay on the AMCAS?

A:
I know how it started because I wrote the beginning once and showed it to somebody just kind of thinking that it was crazy and I shouldn't send it in. And I did. I left it there; they convinced me that it was good. I wrote how — it started off by me writing about when I was really little. And I liked to — when I got in bed at night,

I started to pick a hole in the wallpaper over by my bed. And I went through that layer to see what was next and I kept going through all these layers because I wanted to get all the way out to the stairwell that was on the other side of the wall to see what was inside a wall. So I kind of tied that in with the fact that I've always been sort of interested in how things work. That's how it started.

Q:
That's kind of unusual.

A:
After that, it just kind of got into how I got interested in the things that led me to speech pathology. Like in college, I studied experimental psychology and took a lot of neurology/physiology courses dealing with the brain. I wrote maybe a sentence about that, maybe 2 sentences, and then how that led me to speech pathology. It was kind of tricky because I had to write how that I liked what I was doing and that's what stimulated me to go to medical school, yet I wasn't happy with just doing that, I needed a challenge. I think I used more of a challenge theme for the essay. And I had considered going to medical school right out of college, so I did write that. But at the time I wasn't mature enough, but now I had worked. Now was my time. So that's basically it.

Actually, my boyfriend who does a lot of writing, he read it and edited it for me. Actually, I did a lot of writing in high school, I took AP English and everything. So I always thought I knew how to write. But he showed me all these phrasing mistakes and punctuation mistakes and things like that, so he really cleaned it up for me and helped me to make it short enough so I didn't have to make it really teeny to fit on the page. I do recommend having someone else read it who knows English.

Q:
Now I wanted to talk a little bit about your secondary applications.

A:
The only thing I have to say about the secondary application and actually the whole thing, especially the first one, the AMCAS thing — do it as soon as you can. Get it in the first day that you can. I was three weeks late and for some schools, the delays add up. I applied to Rush. I didn't interview until April and I didn't get in because I didn't have my interview until April. And they told me that if I had interviewed earlier, I probably would have gotten in. I was put on the waiting list.

I think I delayed more on my secondary applications than the first one, because I know I turned in the first one three weeks after the first time you could. But even for that one, I'd get it in the first day. I'm a procrastinator. Don't be a procrastinator.

Q:
Did you recycle some of the essays that you used for one school application and use them on other school applications?

A:
Oh yeah, definitely. Well, I'd use some of the ideas, but change it around.

Q:
How did you choose the different schools that you applied to?

A:
I only applied to a few schools. I knew I wanted to go to school in Chicago. I only applied to schools in Chicago. And actually to Case Western Reserve because my parents live in Cleveland, and they wanted me to go over there.

At first I thought I really wanted to go to U of Illinois just because I had heard that it was a good school. It's also a state school — it's really cheap. I went on a tour there, saw why it was really cheap and didn't want to go there. So I ruled that out. Actually any school where you have to sit in a lecture hall all day, I just can't imagine. That's one reason — probably THE reason why I came to Northwestern. Also I worked across the street so I'm familiar with this place. So basically, I didn't have much strategy in deciding, other than I wanted to come here. And I knew about the schools in the area and the ones I really wanted to go to.

Q:
Did you have professional relationships with physicians at different medical schools in Chicago?

A:
Not really. What I was doing was in the medical field, but I was working — I worked for 2 years in the inpatient facility. And then I was working in this outpatient facility, but it really wasn't very medical. It was sort of like working in a doctor's office, but in those days, the people I was seeing really didn't have very many medical problems, weren't even in wheelchairs. They were getting physical therapy, but all of them could walk at that time. Now it's

completely different. We're getting people who are at a much lower level after their accidents. So even though it was medical, I didn't really have a lot of contacts other than the people at the Rehab. Institute of Chicago.

Q:
This is kind of jumping subjects, but it has to do with recommendations. How did you choose the people to write recommendations for you?

A:
The guy at Loyola helped me figure that out — who you had to have. I think I had 2 of the faculty. You needed three teachers, so I think I used 2 from Loyola and then one could be either from graduate school or undergraduate — it didn't have to be from Loyola. I know I had gotten a really good letter of recommendation from work, from one of my previous professors from the Master's program at Northwestern, the speech pathology program. So I went back to see him and told him what I was doing, and he wrote me a new letter. So I used that.

It really wasn't a problem for me. One of the people on my team who was my direct boss at the RIC program I worked at, we were really more like friends than she was my boss. We used to be equals, then she became the head of the program. She wrote me one — I'm sure it was a really good letter. We worked together for a long time. Then I got one from her boss, my indirect boss, the woman who was the head of the speech department for all of RIC who in a way is sort of my boss also because I'm a speech pathologist. I had know her since 1987. And I know she really liked me. So it was 2 people from work, and 3 academics.

Q:
Tell me a little bit about your interviews. What were the different styles?

A:
I only did two interviews because I got into Northwestern pretty quick and I was pretty sure I wanted to come here. I interviewed here and at Rush. So for Northwestern, the interview was a panel interview. Four people being interviewed and three physicians and a fourth-year medical student.

Sometimes they asked a question to anybody, anybody could answer. Well do I go first, should I be aggressive or whatever? And other times, they directed just specific questions to just one of us. They didn't always ask all four of us the same question, so you couldn't think and formulate an answer while the other people were answering.

I kind of kidded around a little in there. And that was the atmosphere of it. It was really relaxed. The doctors were sort of lounging around, they were not sitting straight up. They had on their gray coats, they didn't have on suits or anything. I was really nervous because it was my first interview, but I still found that I could make a few jokes and things seemed to go over pretty well. I guess it just depends on the feeling of the room.

At Rush, I interviewed with 2 different people, 2 different doctors. I went to the physician's office and waited in the waiting room with his patients and then interviewed in his office at Rush. I kind of liked that. The other guy I met in the library. By then I was more relaxed, I had already gotten in here. I tried to enjoy the interviews. I wasn't quite successful with that here, I was too nervous. At the end, it was OK. Actually at the end of the Northwestern one, I sat in the office shooting the breeze with one of the guys who had been interviewing us about people he knew at RIC.

Q:
Do you have any general advice about interviewing?

A:
I guess my only advice would be just to make sure you get there on time, get a good night's sleep like all the books say and try and be yourself. It's easier to be yourself. You'll be more relaxed than trying to fake it and be someone else. Just be yourself and let your personality shine through.

Q:
You've given a lot of advice. Are there some general recommendations for a student applying now? Things that you think are especially important?

A:
I really think that being a non-traditional student helps you when you get into school. I don't know if it helps you in the application process other than it can help you be more positive about your chances of getting in. And I think I realize now more than I did when I was applying how much it would really help me once I got to school. I don't know if it's going to help me when I'm a doctor, probably, but it's even helped me in school knowing how to get

along with people. Just having more experience out in the world. So, those might be things to mention on the applications or in the interview. It might make you feel better too, just knowing that you're a little older . Even though you might not think so, you can probably handle the interviews a little bit better than some of the people right out of school. I didn't believe that at the time. I thought, oh these people just got out of school, they're probably really sharp. Not that they weren't, but I think that no matter how smart you are and how well you've done in school, just being a little older is going to help you know yourself better. You can relax more and have more to write about on the essay. Just trying to play up what you've done and think about how it relates to what you're going to have to do as a doctor. Think about the different aspects of whatever your career was, not just the obvious things. Also, save your money because you'll need it when you go back to school.

Q:
Good advice, thanks.

Interview Fourteen — Lisa Berg

LISA BERG: Lisa is thirty and married. She graduated from University of Wisconsin at Eau Claire with a Bachelor of Science in Nursing. She then worked as a bone marrow transplant nurse in a number of hospitals.

A:
My name is Lisa Berg and I'm 30 years old. I graduated in 1988. Eau Claire, Wisconsin with a Bachelor of Science in Nursing. I worked full time as a nurse in a variety of hospitals. Also, I did 2 years of traveling nursing across the United States where I work at different hospitals.

Q:
What type of nursing did you do specifically?

A:
I did bone marrow transplant, that's my specialty, but also med surg when I was a traveling nurse. So I worked in different med surg wards.

Q:
I see. And how did you make the decision to go back to medical school?

A:
Well, when I was in nursing school, I thought about going into medical school at that point, but I wasn't quite sure if I would like medicine, so I decided to wait and see how I liked nursing. After a year of nursing, I really enjoyed the patient contact but still realized that I wanted to pursue a higher degree. At that point, I was contemplating nurse practitioner versus MD, so I talked to someone at the Admissions Office at Loyola University School of Medicine. And at that point he said the best thing I could do would be to get a few more years of nursing behind me, to get more experience with medicine, so that's what I did. I ended up working 5 solid years as a nurse. And then I started back on my premed courses at Loyola University.

Q:
So how did you finally decide to make the break and go for it?

A:

It took a lot of thought because I realized that I would be giving up a lot of my free time and maybe even having to postpone family life because I did get engaged at the same time as I started back on my premed courses. But it was a decision that I realized every year I was a nurse that I wanted it more and more. That I knew I wanted to go back.

There were many reasons why I didn't stay in nursing. Let's see if I can name a few. I think the main reason is there's not much of a hierarchy in nursing. You can become a nurse manager and be in charge of a unit or a floor, but that's something that didn't appeal to me because it's more administrative work. You'd be taking care of a budget instead of people and I didn't want to do that. So I thought this was the best option for me in order to maintain patient contact and also increase my autonomy and also have more input into the medical decision making process. I really love that part of it. Deciding what needs to be done, what's going on with the patient and things like that.

Q:

Great. When you went back to school, what type of program did you enroll in?

A:

At Loyola University, they have a program called the post-baccalaureate pre-health program and it's designed for non-traditional students from any background who want to go back and get their medical degree. So I was referred to Dr. Goldman. He's actually no longer there I think. But anyway, that's who was in charge of the program at that time. And he created it. He was a chemistry professor at Loyola and so many people would come up to him and say, how do I get into medical school?

So he created this program that helps you with filling out your medical school applications. He brought back people who had obtained their medical degrees to speak to us in an open forum and tell us what it was like trying to get in, what would be the best thing. The trick you kept on hearing over and over was try and make yourself unusual — stick out among the crowd. That's what they emphasized. He said it was important to get involved in some extracurricular activities, to volunteer at a local hospital or any community center or group. Basically he then said what courses you needed to take.

Q:
What courses did you need? Obviously, you probably had some of them covered from your nursing degree?

A:
Well I did. Actually, the only one I really had covered was biology as an undergrad, but it was 7 years since I had last looked at biology. Actually Dr. Goldman said, why don't you take it over? So I did. I took the whole year of biology over again. And I'm glad I did because there's so much which I had forgotten. And then I had to take inorganic and organic chem and physics.

Q:
When you were studying for your courses, what materials did you find the most helpful? Did you use textbooks, did you use old tests, did you use your notes, study groups, tutors?

A:
I didn't use tutors but they were there if I wanted them. I found that the best way for me was to buy the recommended text and just to read it. Sometimes, I took notes from the text and used that as a review for the exam and I found actually my notes to be the most helpful because that was what was being emphasized in the course.

Q:
Anything else that helped you?

A:
Getting together with some other people from class was helpful because then you sort of found out where you were, what level you were learning the material and what you needed to learn better. And also students make great teachers when they know the material because they can explain it in simpler terms, which helps.

Q:
Which all of us need. Tell me a little bit about the advisement that you received.

A:
Actually not. I basically was told what classes to take. And I just did the applications on my own and really didn't have much help with that. But I didn't find it that difficult. It was just putting in the time and sitting down and thinking about those essay questions.

Q:

Did you participate in extracurricular activities? Obviously, you didn't have to volunteer in a hospital.

A:

I actually did not do extracurricular activities because I was working every weekend as a nurse. And I thought that just keeping up my skill level and also patient contact was the best thing for me to do.

Q:

As far as the MCAT, when did you take it?

A:

I took it in the spring.

Q:

Do you think that's important? The timing? Do you think it's important to take it one time or the other?

A:

I think that if you are done with the course work and you're finishing up your courses in the spring or you're going to finish in May, I think spring is the best time to take it because things are very fresh in your mind. And you've covered 90% of the material. You might be missing 10% that you hadn't finished, but I thought the spring was the best time for me.

Q:

Did you take any review courses?

A:

I took the Kaplan review course. I really didn't find it that helpful. They had these 4 review books that you could work out of, but I found that if you just did well in your classes, your premed classes, that really you learned enough. And just to go back and review your notes from those classes, and that would be enough.

Q:

So that's how you organized your studying? Around your old notes?

A:

Yeah. And then I bought the review book which I found really helpful. Flower's and Barron's.   Also, Kaplan provided questions after every chapter which were very MCAT-like questions, so I utilized that too.

Q:
And how long did you study?

A:
I would say I studied for every weekend for about 2 months and then all of spring Break which was a great time. It was a whole week off and I focused my energies on the MCAT.

Q:
Do you remember your AMCAS application?

A:
I put the things I did in undergrad. Because since I graduated, the only thing I could put was nursing. So I just put activities like Council president, National Residency Hall Honorary, resident assistant, assistant manager while I was in college for a clothing store, Red Cross blood drive volunteer, intramural volleyball and tennis, Special Olympics volunteer, camp counselor. Then I listed all the hospitals I worked at when I was a nurse. When I was traveling, I worked at about 10 major hospitals.

Q:
What did you write your essay about?

A:
Basically, I explained what I was doing the 6 years after I graduated, that I was working full-time as a nurse. And then I talked about my travel nursing, how I chose travel nursing to broaden my experience by working at several institutions. And I talked about my bone marrow transplant experience and how working with cancer patients was the most challenging. Actually, I got into a whole paragraph just about cancer patients. I said that working as a cancer nurse, we were their last hope in their long battle against this devastating disease. They had not only to fight their cancer but also to endure vigorous treatments that themselves were life-threatening. Furthermore, they were confronted with intimidating new technology as well as the prospect that the treatment might fail. I spent much of my time trying to alleviate the anxieties of the patient and family by providing needed encouragement and emotional support. Since these treatments usually entailed numerous and

lengthy hospitalizations, I was able to develop long-term relationships with both patients and family members. This taught me the importance of a trusting care provider relationship which is even more essential in the midst of today's impersonal technology.

Q:
That's good.

A:
I was also exposed to challenging ethical issues such as the right to die with dignity versus the use of heroic life-saving measures. That's was the gist of it.

Q:
On to the secondary applications. How did you use those to your advantage do you think and what was your general impression of them?

A:
Well I found that once you started receiving one after the other, that the questions were basically similar in each one. There might be a slight variation to the same theme of why do you want to go into medicine and why would you be a great doctor? So I felt like if I spent a good amount of time thinking about those 2 questions, that I could come up with an essay that could sort of be used in all of them. So I wasn't just trying to think up original ideas for every application.

Q:
Did you keep them on computer?

A:
Yeah, I kept them on Microsoft Word. That's what I wrote on too, which was great because then you can move things around.

Q:
After the secondary, did you update your application, did you call schools, did you do anything unusual?

A:
I would say after a month later, I called to make sure they received it. Because you always have that fear that they didn't get it. And there's a time limit too and that they have to receive it by this date or that date. So I called to make sure.

Q:
When did you apply?

A:
I actually applied 2 years in a row. I got wait listed the first time I applied. And so I reapplied the second year, so it must have been I applied in '93 and '94.

Q:
As far as timing, did you get your applications out early?

A:
Yes, and I think that helped the second time.   The first time I was sort of late. The second time, I made sure I had it them by the earliest date and turned around secondaries within a week.
Another thing about answering the essay question that I think is good to do is be creative. The first time I applied, there was this question — it was pick from the list of adjectives which one describes you. Okay, so you could pick organized, ambitious, and so on. If you get questions like that, try and be creative with it, with any question really. What I ended up doing is I made an acronym with all the letters and I spelled out something.

Q:
That's great! What was it, do you remember?

A:
I spelled out, it's really corny, I'm embarrassed to say. But you never know — they might have looked at it and said, gosh, look at this. I made it funny because I sort of laughed at it. The acronym was "a good person." And I used words that started with each of those letters.

Q:
That is creative! Those things can be so dry.

A:
I think these people who read these applications can fall asleep after a while. So I think they appreciate any type of humor and creativity that someone throws in.

Q:
I'm sure they do, reading 10,000 boring essays.

A:

And plus too, you're going to stick out. Another way to stick out from the crowd.

Q:

You seem to really think that's important, to make yourself seen.

A:

I do. When you're talking an average of 9-10,000 applications per school, that is a heck of a lot of applications. Everybody is going to have an excellent academic record and pretty good MCAT scores, so it really comes down to your essay and your extracurricular activities.

Q:

How many schools did you end up applying to?

A:

I applied to ten. I was restricted with my husband in applying to only 2 cities, Chicago and Boston. All of Chicago and all of Boston.

Q:

That's a good number of schools.

A:

I was lucky that I had the choice — not many cities support 6 schools like Chicago.

Q:

As far as your recommendations went, how did you choose the people you got recommendations from?

A:

I really tried to play up my nursing background. I think if you have any type of experience in the medical field, definitely play that up. So I chose a physician I had worked with and my nurse manager.

Q:

How about your academic recommendations?

A:

Because I was out of school for 7 years, I was limited. I had to use references from Loyola where I did my premed. So I asked my biology teacher and my organic chem teacher to do a reference.

Q:
Why did you choose them over the other ones?

A:
I felt like I had a better rapport. I made a point that they knew who I was. I would go into their office periodically and make sure they knew me by first name. And that way when I knew it was time to get a reference, they'd say yeah, Lisa, Okay. And they knew who I was.

Q:
On to your interviews. Tell me basically your general impression of your interviews, and the different types, the different questions that you remembered, liked or disliked. And how did you prepare — did you prepare?

A:
Yeah. Actually the program at Loyola gave us a bunch of handouts that were to facilitate your preparing for your interview. So it was a bunch of mock questions. And I had my husband read the questions to me and then I ad libbed it. So that way I was sort of organizing my thoughts in my head before I went in. And I did this a day or two before the interview. Just went through them. Because you don't want to sound programmed either when you talk.

Q:
Do you remember any specifics? Any ethical questions?

A:
I remember at Rush Medical School, there was a question that sort of turned into a heated debate and I felt like it sort of might have hindered me getting in. And it was about — we were talking about tube-feeding for people who are terminally ill. Basically I was telling the interviewer my view about it, how it can sort of prolong life.

Q:
You might have had more experience than they did.

A:
I don't even know if the interviewer was an MD. I think he was just an administrator head. He wanted me on the spot to say yes or no if I would stop the tube feedings. And I just couldn't tell him yes or no, because I said, well it depends on the circumstances, it

depends on the patient's family, if there are other medical conditions and everything. But he said, no, I was being evasive. I needed to make the decision. So that was sort of hard, I felt.

Q:
I think lots of times they just challenge you just to see if you'll back down.

A:
Yeah, maybe he was just trying to see if I would wax and wane.

Q:
Anything else that you remember from your interviews?

A:
I've heard horror stories about other peoples' interviews. Mine went basically well. I felt the questions were very fair. Actually at the other interviews, I didn't have any ethical, really right-to-die issues brought up. I felt like they were pretty fair and what you would expect from an interview.

Q:
So just trying to get to know you?

A:
Yeah. Like what have you done the last five years? What's your experience? Why do you want to go into medicine?

Q:
Or why do you want to change what you're doing?

A:
Exactly. Why do you want to change? Why don't you like nursing?

Q:
How did you answer that one, if they said why don't you like nursing?

A:
Well, I told them that I love nursing. And it's definitely something that's going to be hard for me to give up as a career. It has a great many perks. It's a great career. But then I went into my reasons that I gave before — just having more independence, I want to

learn more about the pathophysiological basis of disease. That's
something that in nursing we skimmed over. We never learned
hard core medicine. As a nurse our scientific knowledge, our medical knowledge is limited, and it's based mainly on experience. A
new grad doesn't know much. But you ask a ten-year veteran nurse
, and she knows a lot based on experience.

Q:
Do you have any general recommendations?

A:
I think the most important decision for applicants to make is do
they want to sacrifice a good seven years of their life to undergo
rigorous training and education. That's the most important decision. Make sure that this is what you want to do. And I would recommend getting volunteer experience in a hospital. Hospitals are
always looking for volunteers. I think having a career before you
go into medicine, whatever field it's in, I think it's a definite asset.
Play it up and be proud of your background and what you've done
before you go into medicine.

Also applying to medical school as a nurse has its advantages, because they know what they're getting into. That's what
everybody at work says. Like all these doctors that I talk to. And I
say, oh, I'm going back. And the doctors say, at least you know
what to expect. Because they say, I didn't. And it's a shock — it
could be a definite shock. Like I said, I've been on the other side
of the bed. As a nurse. The other side.

Q:
Thanks a lot Lisa.

Interview Fifteen — Michelle Montpetit

MICHELLE MONTPETIT: Michelle is a twenty six years old. She graduated from Drake University with a degree in Pharmacy and worked as a in-patient pharmacist at Northwestern hospital before applying to medical school. She continues to work during medical school as time permits.

A:
My name is Michelle Montpetit and I'm 27.

Q:
Tell me a little bit about what you did before you came to medical school.

A:
Okay, I graduated from Drake University with a BS in Pharmacy and an emphasis in business in 1992. I worked at Northwestern Memorial Hospital for 3 years prior to going to medical school. At Northwestern, I was actively involved in patient care, developing therapeutic regimens, working directly with the residents and the house staff to determine the best regimen for patient care. In addition, we had responsibilities that included dispensing and active teaching roles where we would provide classes to nursing, other pharmacists and house staff. A lot of activities.

Q:
How did you make the decision to go back to medical school?

A:
Actually I joined the staff of Northwestern with the idea of becoming a physician anyway. They offered the position to me when I was here as a pharmacy student and at the time, they knew I was considering medical school. And they said they'd give me a year to figure out if I wanted to be a physician or a pharmacist. And to take my prerequisites for medical school and to just learn a little bit about life and pharmacy.

But my actual decision — I made my decision when I was a 4th year pharmacy student. I was doing an internship at Walgreen's and realized that I was working very hard at a degree that didn't provide a lot of job satisfaction in the real world. The emphasis was on making money and not patient care. Although I think Walgreen's pharmacists do provide patient care in some settings, it was just dispensing. There was no clinical interaction, and in school we were being taught that the world of pharmacy was leaning toward a very clinically-oriented very proactive career that we would be actively involved in patient care. And that wasn't my experience at Walgreen's.

At that time, I decided — I was working on my degree in pharmacy and my MBA— and so what I did was drop the MBA program. I didn't really enjoy business anyway, and I picked up a minor in biology. So when I graduated, I had a BS in pharmacy with a minor in biology as well. I had the support of many of the PhDs in the pharmacy program. I think they realized that I'd probably always want something else other than pharmacy.

I was wrong though. I went to Northwestern and it's a great set-up for a pharmacist. I put my education to work daily. I thought that it was a wonderful place to work. It was hard to decide once I was accepted to medical school which way to go just because I did have a career that I enjoyed a lot. But that's not the real world of pharmacy and I'd probably be very limited in my practice options.

Q:
O.K. Tell me a little bit about your premed courses and how you went about taking them.

A:
Fortunately most of the premed courses were incorporated in my undergraduate degree as a pharmacist. The only thing I was lacking was a year of physics. So I had plenty of schools in the area that I could choose. I chose Loyola because they did have a post-bacc program which facilitated classes in the evening core. It facilitated the core medical — the premed courses during the summer and evening hours.

Q:
So that was important for you? The flexibility?

A:
Yeah, I worked shifts. So we would work 3 weeks of a day shift which was 7:30-4:00 and we'd work one week of evenings. So during the duration of the physics course that I took, I would either not be able to be work those evenings or have to adjust my schedule. So that means it would involve all the people that I work with. So what I did was I took the first physics course during the summer at Loyola and I worked all evenings. And I went to school all morn-

ing and then I'd come back and I'd work all evening. But it was a very limited time that we were doing that. I think I was only in school for about 4 weeks total. And it was nice to take an entire semester of physics in 4 weeks. It was a lot of work, but on the other hand it was just very concise and provided all the information I needed for the MCAT.

The second physics course I took during the spring semester a year later. And again, the way they had the course set up, there was no difference between the summer and the year program. They covered the same material. They're very helpful and accommodating to people who work and are going to school.

Q:
What premedical courses did you cover during pharmacy school?

A:
Well I had a semester of biochemistry, a semester of medicinal chemistry. I had a year of inorganic, a year of organic, biochemistry, medical chemistry. I had a year of physiology. I had a pathophysiology course. I had a full microbiology course. I had 2 years of pharmacotherapeutics. I had 2 years of pharmaceutics. I had one semester of pharmacokinetics, one semester of biopharmacodynamics, which is kinetics in the body applied directly to the patient and specific agents.

Also, I had my Biology II course which was an anatomy course of sorts; we studied human anatomy but we dissected a cat. So it was important to have some idea of, just because for medical terminology's sake if nothing else. So between the second semester of biology and the physiology, it kind of all comes together.

Q:
So you had extensive premedical courses?

A:
Yeah. And I had neuropharm and neuropysch and neurophysiology.

Q:
That's fantastic. Tell me a little bit about your advisement. Who did you use for planning your post-bacc, and tell me a little bit about the people that you used to advise you for the application process.

A:
For the application process or even for just the post-bacc, I con-

sulted the people from Drake University, from my undergraduate program, quite a bit. Most of them had PhDs in pharmacology. I had worked closely with one gentleman while I was doing research and he had worked closely with many — he had at one point applied to medical school but decided that he wanted to get his Ph.D. instead. In addition, he had worked with many professors at Texas Tech medical school, so he had a lot of information for me. And he had a lot of people to consult. There was a premed committee at Drake and I consulted the head of the committee on occasion, but I also used other members just to talk and clarify my questions. And so although I wasn't guided through the premed process like a lot of the biology majors were, I knew those professors well enough so that going back and being away from Drake, I could still call and ask questions. So I just used the resources that had been available to me.

Q:
How about your professional contacts?

A:
I had help with writing my personal statement. I kind of took polls on who had taken the Kaplan course. For the material like Kaplan and reading my personal statement, I utilized many of the residents and the house staff. And other med students — I worked closely with them. They all provided their own experiences. Personal statements and letters of reference, I had many of the attendings who work at Northwestern provide letters.

Q:
Okay, we'll get a little more into that later. As far as extracurricular activities, your career was in medicine, so did you do other activities that were medically-related during your application process or before?

A:
I was very involved while I was in pharmacy school. I was on the Dean's Advisory Committee. I was a member of the Alumni Association for the university. I was involved with a professional pharmacy fraternity which did a great deal of philanthropy work. When I was in Chicago, I did a lot. I was involved in the American Society of Hospital Pharmacists.

I was getting hands-on experience at work as far as from the medicine perspective. I went on rounds daily and so I was getting that experience. What I did do was I went to homeless shelters and volunteered there working with kids who were disadvantaged. Depending on how long I was there or how many times during the week that I went, I'd either provide tutorials, opportunities to read one-on-one or play games depending on the age of the children involved during the night. Reading or playing, singing songs. If they're preschool, we typically played or had story time. If they were older children, then I would provide them with tutoring.

Q:
As far as giving advice to someone who's in the application process, do you think the extracurriculars make a big difference, and what ones would you recommend?

A:
Well, I think it is important that you show that you're involved — they want physicians who are involved in the community and people who are going to give back. Because although we provide care and a lot of our time's not going to be our own, they still want people who are able to balance many activities and do them all very well.

I think it is important to be involved. I think it's important to volunteer at a hospital or something, just to get an idea of what it's like to be around patients.   Hospice programs are wonderful because you really get a unique experience dealing with family and friends. I think emergency rooms — I'm not sure that, in general, hospital volunteer experiences are considered that wonderful just because you're not always dealing directly with patients. But if you can demonstrate that you spent time talking to the patient and their family, experiences you've gained, I think it is valuable. And I think it helps you realize what's expected of you as a physician. I think volunteer experience is important and also taking leadership roles. I also took call while I was a pharmacist.   I had took the opportunity to take call.   Oftentimes, if you know somebody who's involved in medicine, they can help secure a position like that. Because that was strictly voluntary.

Q:
Taking call, meaning spending the night at the hospital and seeing patients with a resident?

A:
Yeah. I took a couple of Friday and Saturday nights. I'd go up from work directly to the floor and spend the entire night running around

with them, going to micro lab and hematology to look at smears because there was no one else to give a final say so.   It's a good experience.

Q:
Now we're going to move on to the MCAT. First of all, when did you take it?

A:
The first time I took the MCAT was September of 1991. And I took it without taking physics. I did Okay, I didn't do well. I was advised when I was applying that it would look better if I took it again just to show some improvement — I had been wait listed at one school and I was waiting to hear from Northwestern. I was advised to just take it again. So I took it again and I subsequently improved some of the scores, and it worked out obviously.

Q:
So that was in '91. Did you apply then also?

A:
I applied and I was accepted to a program contingent on taking physics. And that was the year that I was going to graduate from college. And Northwestern had already offered the position and I had already accepted it.

Q:
You decided to take your pharmacy position?

A:
Right, instead of going to medical school right away. I knew that it was going to take an entire summer to take physics anyway. So I went ahead and accepted the position at Northwestern, gave up the slot at the State University which had offered me the position. And I took physics. And then I took the MCAT again in April of 1995. It was kind of a waste at that point because I found out soon after that I'd been accepted anyway without the scores. The scores weren't that significantly better, but they were better.

Q:
Well they made you feel better.

A:
Yeah, a little.

Q:
The 2 times you took it, what were your different strategies in studying for it?

A:
Well the first time, I didn't study. I was going into my clinical experience for pharmacy school and I had been doing an internship at a hospital where I was gaining a lot of clinical experience. Although I knew I wanted to go to medical school, I knew I still had to take physics, so it was kind of like a last-minute— I should just take it to see how it goes. And I did and I couldn't be too upset about the scores considering I never really applied myself. The second time around, I used the Flowers book but I didn't use it a lot — again,, I just don't like to study for these standardized tests. And I felt like the MCAT was just a very poor assessment of who I was. So if I were to say that I studied a great deal or prepared about the MCAT, I'd be lying. I didn't.

Q:
But your background is very different.

A:
Right. If I had it to do it over again, I would probably still take — I would take the MCAT possibly the spring a year before I wanted to go to medical school. I hear strong accolades for the Kaplan course and some of the other courses that are available. So I think that if I were to do it again, I would consider either taking it over a year before I needed the score, see how I did and consider taking a course such as the Kaplan course, and then taking it again. I would take it at least a year in advance so I had opportunity to improve my scores.

Q:
So the length of time that you studied for it was..?

A:
The first time I didn't study for it. The second time that I took it I studied casually for a month before and then 2 weeks before I really made an effort to go through some of the questions. That's what I did for the most part — kind of went through questions.

Q:
Did you do the old tests that were available?

A:

I did one of them. And I still didn't do them like — they recommend that you do them as though you're taking an exam, but I didn't do it that way. I think it's more important to just read and get an idea of the question. A lot of it's just test-taking. A lot of it's problems, what they call problem-solving skills. That's more intuitive.

Q:

On to the AMCAS application.   How did you choose what do put on there and what to leave off? What did you try to emphasize?

A:

I tried to emphasize my leadership roles. Obviously, just grades and whatnot, I just threw that stuff on. But everything else, I tried to show that I was very involved. That throughout the time I was in school, I was not only in the community, but I was involved in my profession and I was involved with fun activities. I just had good balance, and that is what I thought was most important. Leadership, balance.

Q:

And for your essay, what did you write about?

A:

I wrote about my experiences that would lead me to go to medical school. And I really didn't use a lot of my pharmacy background. I talked about it at the end in saying that I had a good idea of what I was about to get into. I looked at different experiences I had in school. First I listed 3 things that I thought were key to being a physician and 3 things that I wanted to do with it.

Q:

What were those?

A:

Educate, be a caretaker and provider.   It was really about just being there to listen, to provide care and to educate. And I tied in my pharmacy background with the fact that that was part of the reason why I was leaving, that I wasn't allowed to provide a lot of one-on-one care. I think I discussed my volunteer experience here in Chicago and the teaching I did.

Q:

Which volunteer experience?

A:

The one with the kids where I would go and tutor. And how I had
to separate myself, how I had to learn to be — because they were
coming from backgrounds that I would never understand by being
in their shoes — but I'd have to accept and not criticize or be judgmental because we do face people everyday that we have no idea
what is going on and when you know, it's hard sometimes not to
just accept it. But I learned how to have a professional goal, and
just accept what's there and try to make what time I had with them
good. And that's the sort of thing I emphasized.

Q:

Was there anything you wanted to add about your essay?

A:

I just emphasized what characteristics I had and what I wanted to
provide as a doctor. And how the experiences I had in the past
helped me just learn that being a physician is what I want more
than anything else at this time.

Q:

Now we're going to talk about your secondary applications. What
was your general impression and how did you try to use them to
your advantage?

A:

The state schools are generally very quick and easy. They don't ask
a lot of questions and it's kind of annoying. Although you look at
the ones with all the essays and you're like, oh god. But the thing
is I noticed in my interviews that they really did read those. And
the state schools— I just felt like they didn't have a sense of who I
was or what I was. Everything they had was from the AMCAS,
which is fine, but again, someone with experience, it's limited. So
this gave me the opportunity to expound.

Q:

In additional essays?

A:

The essays, yeah. They're kind of a pain to write, but it really let me
say, why did I want a certain program? Well, again I was fortunate
to work with many residents, many different programs. So let's say
that I were interested in Vermont's program. I could talk to a resident who's from that program and I was able to say, well, on the

plus side this is what your program could provide me. That program I think is especially geared toward non-traditionals.   And so I really was able to look at it.

And working at Northwestern, I was very aware of the new curriculum, the problem-based learning. And although they advertise it, I was able to discuss this regularly with students. I knew what I thought the advantages were and I also knew the limitations of such a program and I noted that how I saw there were limitations, but that I could adjust , that your education is what you make of it, and you can express that. For the essays I think it's just as . important to have several people read them and give their opinion. And people from very different parts of your life. Not just your friends, but maybe somebody you've worked with or a professor. Just say, please just assess this critically. Tell me what your impression was when you read it. And I found that very helpful.

Q:
When did you apply?

A:
I started my applications in August. I had my AMCAS ready to go by mid-August and I sent that out, and so I received secondaries quite early. Just because of the sheer numbers of people applying, it does take a long time. I didn't hear from some programs to be offered interviews until January or February. And I just had to be calm. And they say, well in the past we've filled our class by March so if you haven't heard from us, that's a bad sign. And when I was applying, most of the programs I talked to said, well you haven't heard from us, but that doesn't mean anything because we're just so overwhelmed with volume. And it did. I was still being offered interviews later on, late January when I thought it was rather late to be interviewing, especially for having early applications in.

Q:
How many schools did you apply to?

A:
I applied to nine. Three dream schools, three good programs that I was very interested in and three sure-things, so to speak. And that's how I selected them. I just kind of went through. I really didn't care where I ended up so as far as geographics, it didn't matter. And I just applied to programs that I thought I was very interested in based on the Medical School Admission Requirements book by AMCAS. I just had a number of schools I was interested in. And

again, I was able to talk to residents and attendings. I knew what programs they were from.

Q:
That's a big advantage.
A:
It certainly was. I was fortunate to have the inside scoop on most programs. And people that knew people at other schools.

Q:
Your recommendations, how did you choose the people that you had write recommendations for you?

A:
Well, they usually ask for three professors or your premed committee. Again, I didn't utilize the premed committee. My program was very heavy in the sciences. I think it's good to get a balance of professors. Twenty percent of my education was liberal arts. But I didn't feel that those professors really knew who I was, and my science professors did. So I did end up using three science professors for my recommendations.

Q:
So which one's did you select?

A:
The man I did research with. My physiology professor because when I first started taking his course, I don't think I knew how to study and approach physiology. And I went to talk to him, because I wasn't doing well academically at all. One of my professors, Dr. Statton, kind of sat me down and said, you just don't know what you're doing. You just don't know the material. He taught me how to apply everything and learn concept, not just learn the material. Because obviously if you just try and memorize and know the material by rote, you'll never be able to apply it. After the third exam, I got a 100%, and Stratton's like, oh, you took my advice. And I took another course with him and I did very well. I thought that he really knew me. He saw me struggling and for somebody like me to struggle academically was pretty unusual. It was really hard.

Anyway, I chose the guy I did research with, a man that had seen me really grow academically, learn how to think intellectually, and another professor who's just a friend. The infectious disease pharmacist was somebody who I think was very well aware of my talents, what I had to offer to the department. And he had asked me to teach a course on general medicine and the pharmacist. And so I thought, he certainly knows me. I had him write one and I had one of the medicine attendings write one.

Q:
For most of your science classes, how did you study? What did you use? Did you use textbooks, did you use old tests, notes? And how did you do it before this transition in this one class and how did you do it afterwards?

A:
I always used my notes. I would go to books on occasion. Fortunately for me, the transition occurred in the very beginning of my third year of pharmacy school. And the first two years are again core curriculum basic science courses — organic, inorganic, biology. The stuff you can get by with just memorizing.

Q:
So the premed courses?

A:
Right. But I used my notes, for the most part. Occasionally, I'd study with a partner. I never was a big group study person but I did have one person I would study with regularly for the basic sciences.

For the pharmacy curriculum, I always would study my notes and I would read occasionally. But we were fortunate to have really good syllabi. So they really provided us a lot of detail and you just had to go over it a couple of times, have an idea. I would often times, especially for physiology, do the review questions that were provided. Because I had never done them before and I obviously had to do everything that could possibly pull me out of my tailspin that I was in. And I did. I did the review questions and I learned all of sudden that those objectives were there for a reason. I really had always gotten by — things came very easily.

And then for some of the pharmacy courses, for therapeutics courses though, the stuff that was physiology-applied and pharmacology, there were no test files. Tests weren't available — it was always a closed exam. For pharmaceutics, I used questions but there weren't just a lot of exams available for physiology.

Q:
So what did you use?

A:
My notes.

Q:
How about textbooks?

A:
I'm not a textbook reader. If I didn't understand something from my notes and my colleagues were in a similar situation, then I would read the textbook. I would just clarify any details that I needed. And I still don't like to study from textbooks.

Q:
Now we're going to talk a little bit about your interviews. Tell me the different styles of interviews you had.

A:
I had one-on-one interviews. I've had two interviewers and myself. I've had panel interviews. I think the absolute worst is the panel. I didn't like three students with three faculty members. Because inevitably you get some bozo who thinks they're just ready to talk talk talk and just very inflated self-esteem. And it's like, all right, whatever, I'm a very confident person. But I don't want to listen to somebody just go on and on for no reason. I didn't like the panel. But I've had one-on-one, two-on-one and panel. I definitely liked the one-on-one.

Q:
Do you remember any questions that you liked or disliked?

A:
It was funny. In a couple of interviews, I was hit with a lot of ethical questions. I enjoyed them, but I was hit with quite a few of them. Especially with the pharmacy industry and the drug companies and what they provide physicians. I was asked a lot of questions about that. And I was already very opinionated, so it kind of hit my — well, I think all the marketing is a terrible waste of money. They got a good laugh out of it. I always tried to relax.

I enjoyed it when they asked me about, kind of get an idea of what I knew about what was going on in the world today. Questions about stress I think are important questions that they ask and how you manage stress. And you may wonder why or what they're trying to get at or think it's a stupid question. But they need to know if you're going to be able to handle a program and be able to relieve stress. Can you do it just by taking some time alone and thinking? Can you just get by or are you somebody that has to go running or exercise? And if you're not able to, does that just drive you crazy? That's going to be very tough for you in a residency setting. And I didn't understand those questions until I talked to some people who were involved in asking them. And the sort of answers they were looking for.

Q:
Did you do any preparations for your interviews?

A:
One of attendings offered to ask questions. They offered to ask questions and I just didn't want to. I'd rather go into it cold. I tend to interview well. At that point, for me, I would just rather face what I have to face and do it and go through it. It's important I think the night before your interviews to review your personal statement, review your application, read a newspaper, watch the news. I think it's important to read a newspaper. I read the newspaper daily, but I always make sure that I pretty much know what's going on, even in the local towns, because they want to know that you take an interest in life, I think.

   I would just try and relax and go in there very casual. I did have one interview, it wasn't for medical school, it was for a doctor of pharmacy program, but I think it still applies. It was a 12-hour interview. It was the best interview I've ever had though, which is surprising. I didn't prepare, I didn't even try to prepare. And I had actually arrived in the city at 5 o'clock in the morning the day of the interview after traveling for 12 hours on a train. And the one thing I can say is I didn't try and prepare. I went in and I knew who I was and what I was doing and why I was doing it. And I was very comfortable with my decision. It was good interview. I think that's the most important thing. Know who you are and what you want.

Q:
That's great. And then how did you choose the school that you accepted?

A:
Well, I knew I wanted to go to Northwestern. So when I was in, it

was kind of just a done deal. And I think I was most impressed with their program and that was an important factor in why I chose this school. It had to be a competitive program nationwide. A good program. But then I wanted to know how do the students interact with each other? Is it an incredibly competitive environment in which I'd be miserable? And was it someplace that I could still continue to have a good lifestyle? And I think Northwestern's pass/fail system was very attractive. And that really says something for the students too because we work together as teams. And people aren't constantly stressed out. I wanted to be able to have a social life and not always feel that I had to be studying or that all of my classmates were always studying. So those were the sort of things. A school where they promoted balance. Where academic competition — they're all bright students. You have to be bright to get here in the first place. So that's why I chose this school.

Q:
Do you have any general recommendations to someone who's applying to medical school as a non-traditional student?

A:
Utilize your contacts. If you don't get in right away and you really want to be in a certain program, sell yourself. You've done it to an employer already. And don't forget that — it's likely that you had to sell yourself in the past. And remember that you offer them as much as they can offer you. And you just let them know what you can apply to their program, what you could provide. Be in contact with them, let them know how interested you are. And always be professional. I think formal letters are important. And you can be in contact with them but just remember that you have to sell yourself and part of that is saying, I'm professional, I'm mature, this is me. And I think they respect that.

Q:
Good advice to conclude with. Thanks Michelle.

Conclusion

This book has let you see into the lives of the individuals who were interviewed about their time of application to medical school. This book is just a starting point. There are many different resources — many have been mentioned in this book — which will help you on your journey toward medical school. Use as many of them as possible.

As of the printing of this book all of the individuals interviewed are entering their second or third year of medical school. This statement is significant for two reasons. First, all of these non-traditional students got into medical school. There is hope! Second, each of these students were able to make the transition from being a non-traditional premed student to being a successful medical student. Each of these non-traditional students were able to compete successfully with traditional students in the classroom. And their other abilities gained from life experience allowed them to maintain a balanced perspective on the medical school experience.

Another point in closing to discuss takes anyone thinking about applying to medical school back to the start of the process- MAKING THE DECISION. The process of taking premedical classes and completing the application process takes considerable time and effort. However, when compared with four years of medical school and an average four year residency, the application process is not nearly as difficult. For both emotional and financial reasons, make sure that you want to be a physician.

After you are comfortable with your decision to pursue medicine I say "good luck- believe in yourself and you can do it!" The light at the end of the tunnel can be the most emotionally gratifying career on earth.

UP FOR GRABS

Inquiries into Who Wants What